ASSISTED LIVING

FOR OUR PARENTS

A VOLUME IN THE SERIES

The Culture and Politics of Health Care Work

edited by SUZANNE GORDON AND SIOBAN NELSON

From Silence to Voice: What Nurses Know and Must Communicate to the Public, Second Edition
  by BERNICE BURESH AND SUZANNE GORDON

Nobody's Home: Candid Reflections of a Nursing Home Aide
  by THOMAS EDWARD GASS

Nursing against the Odds: How Health Care Cost Cutting, Media Stereotypes, and Medical Hubris Undermine Nurses and Patient Care
  by SUZANNE GORDON

The Complexities of Care: Nursing Reconsidered
  edited by SUZANNE GORDON AND SIOBAN NELSON

Nurses on the Move: Migration and the Global Health Care Economy
  by MIREILLE KINGMA

Code Green: Money-Driven Hospitals and the Dismantling of Nursing
  by DANA WEINBERG

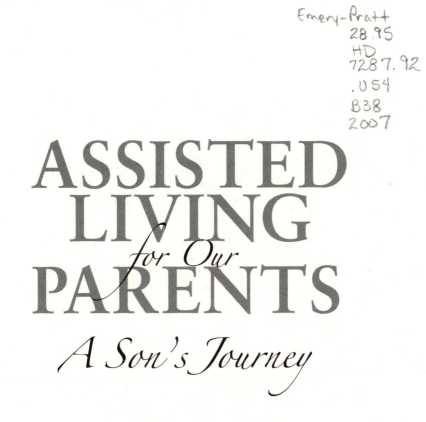

ASSISTED LIVING *for Our* PARENTS

A Son's Journey

DANIEL JAY BAUM

FOREWORD BY CAROL LEVINE

ILR PRESS

an imprint of Cornell University Press

ITHACA AND LONDON

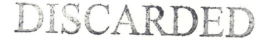

First published 2007 by Cornell University Press

Printed in the United States of America

Library of Congress Cataloging-in-Publication Data

Baum, Daniel Jay.
   Assisted living for our parents : a son's journey / Daniel Jay Baum ; with a foreword by Carol Levine.
      p. cm. — (The culture and politics of health care work)
   Includes bibliographical references and index.
   ISBN-13: 978-0-8014-4468-5 (cloth : alk. paper)
   1. Baum, Ida Frieman. 2. Baum, Daniel Jay. 3. Congregate housing—United States—Case studies. 4. Aging parents—United States—Family relationships—Case studies. 5. Adult children—United States—Family relationships—Case studies. 6. Parent and adult child—United States—Case studies. I. Title. II. Series.
   HD7287.92.U54B38 2007
   362.6'3—dc22   2006035653

Cornell University Press strives to use environmentally responsible suppliers and materials to the fullest extent possible in the publishing of its books. Such materials include vegetable-based, low-VOC inks and acid-free papers that are recycled, totally chlorine-free, or partly composed of nonwood fibers. For further information, visit our website at www.cornellpress.cornell.edu.

Cloth printing   10 9 8 7 6 5 4 3 2 1

For my mother,
Ida Frieman Baum

עֵץ חַיִּים הִיא

She is a Tree of Life.

Contents

Foreword

Today, as millions of North Americans enter midlife and even reach the point of retirement themselves, they grapple with questions such as: Can Mom continue to manage on her own? Is she safe? Should Dad move in with me? What are my obligations to my elderly parents? Those approaching old age also worry about what will happen to them when they themselves cross the age threshold, especially if they are childless. Who will take care of me? Will I have enough money to take care of myself? Will I end up poor and in a nursing home? What can I do now to prevent that?

In this book Daniel Baum, who himself is in his seventies, writes about assisted living facilities, or ALFs—continuing care retirement facilities that numbered over 32,000 in the United States in 2000. He explains what it is like to see one's parent grow old as one also ages. He describes in moving and compelling detail the decision he and his 89-year-old mother, Ida, made to sell her home and move her to an assisted living facility, where she spent her final years.

At first, money didn't appear to be a significant issue. Daniel Baum had a loving relationship with his mother, and as the sole surviving child, he did not have to contend with the dissension and recriminations that are so common among family members as they try to figure out who will take care of Mom and Dad. In addition to being a loving son who wanted to do right by his mother, he is also a lawyer with experience negotiating complex contracts, as well as an academic who has published two books on the nursing home industry and retirement.

In many ways, this story parallels that of thousands of North Americans. In my work at the United Hospital Fund directing a research project on family caregivers, I hear stories every day from daughters, sons, and spouses desperately trying to deal with the latest crisis, sometimes in their own households but often from afar, and almost always with inadequate information. Sometimes I imagine airplanes filled with anguished family caregivers crisscrossing the country to deal with Mom's fall, Dad's erratic driving, the home-care worker's unreliability, or the nursing home's neglect. A special fare for caregivers would be a very good thing.

Policymakers sometimes portray older people and their family members as greedy devourers of public resources; in my experience, the opposite is true. Older people carefully guard their independence and often refuse help of any kind until a disaster forces a change. Adult children must contend with anxiety about maintaining the balance between their parents' autonomy and safety, as well as the safety of others.

Given this state of almost perpetual worry, it is no wonder that families who can afford it see assisted living facilities as a solution and that assisted living facilities market themselves to adult children—the Daniel Baums of the world—with a very particular pitch. A random sampling of web-based descriptions reveals fulsome descriptions of amenities: an "elegant lobby," a "charming dining room," "beautiful views," "superb food." Activities emphasize active participation in sports, crafts, and intellectual discussions. Dedication to "healthy living into high old age" stops just short of promising eternal life. Both adult children and their parents may be particularly attracted by promises of "aging in place," which has become a catch-all concept for a wide variety of living situations that relate to residents' autonomy and independence. As Daniel Baum illustrates, these promises may be hard to fulfill. Assisted living facilities require compromises and accommodations, some necessary, others more for the benefit of management.

The author's journey also reveals the underlying tensions that drive practice and policies in the aging field. There is no single definition for assisted living. Facilities call themselves independent living, continuing care communities, naturally occurring retirement communities, and many other designations. Each state regulates (or doesn't) assisted living differently; to avoid complex skilled nursing home regulations, assisted living facilities and their counterparts distance themselves from the kind of services nursing homes provide.

As he tells the story of his mother's decline and the assisted living facility's response to it, Daniel Baum is questioning, to be sure, while acknowledging its perspective. He understands that all institutions have to protect their own interests to survive. Assisted living facilities also have to protect what they see as the interests of all the residents while at the same time promising each individual independence and autonomy. The author also questions himself. He asks, How could I, a law professor, not have read and appreciated the fine points of the contract? What more could I have done to preserve my mother's independence when she was moved to the skilled nursing facility?

In the story, the reader comes to see just how easily a lawyer or anyone one else can overlook such fine print and readily accept the assurances of assisted living facility administrators during tours and informational interviews. In fact, it is common for gifted professionals in their own right to be unable to transfer their skills and knowledge to the Byzantine world of long-term care when it comes to their own parent or spouse. As I speak to professional groups around the country, I hear many emotional, often angry, stories of how a nurse, social worker, doctor, or lawyer finds the system he or she works in every day unresponsive to his or her own parents' or relatives' needs.

The author asks, Is there a better way? His mother's experience has led him to consider carefully what he wants for himself as he ages and to organize his life to make it happen. For now, he has found an answer for himself in what he describes as his vertical neighborhood, a high-rise complex in downtown Toronto, a mixed-generation facility with amenities and security going far beyond most assisted living facilities. Many of us are looking for solutions, too. It is important for individuals to consider the possibilities realistically. Yet the future may depend on political will and public support for a range of affordable options for long-term care.

Daniel Baum's generous sharing of his experience provides insights and information that will be extremely valuable for many adult children. A careful reading of this book will help them make, if not the best, at least the most informed choice possible for themselves and their parents.

CAROL LEVINE

United Hospital Fund
New York City, September 2006

Acknowledgments

Never before have I written a book in the first person. With my other books, including those on retirement and the nursing home industry, the discipline of academia compelled a certain distance, a sign of objectivity. This book, however, is personal. It reflects the specific experiences of my mother and me.

Without the encouragement, ongoing critique, and specific editorial suggestions from my long-time associate, Penny Mallette, who was also a friend to my mother and me, I doubt that the book would have been completed.

It took more than a few years to find the proper voice, one that is my own. Without Jessica Starr's early help, and that of Lynn Wasnak, friend to both my mother and me, I am not sure that voice would have matured as it did.

I confess to a certain anger when I first considered writing the book. No doubt, some of that anger reflected grief at the loss of my mother. But, some of that anger reflected the institutional nature of assisted living. It took patience and ongoing dialogue with my series editor, Suzanne Gordon, for me to temper the angry edge and achieve a resulting balance. I am grateful for this.

Though this book is a thin volume, several years have been invested in its development. It is, in one sense, the story of my mother. But, in a larger sense, it is not a memoir. I have written it to assist others—adult children trying to help their parents (usually their mothers), and also ourselves, recognizing that we follow in their wake.

I do not claim to be an expert in the several professional fields touched upon in this book. Concern for my mother's ongoing health and safety, her quality of life and, as it turned out, the choices that might have been hers were subjects that I probed. I am not a medical doctor, a specialist in assisted living for the elderly, or one who leads efforts to find alternative living arrangements for the elderly, including independent living. I have my own experience—and that of my mother. Also, I have called on professionals with hands-on practice to review my reasoning and conclusions. Of course, I alone am responsible for the conclusions stated.

Among the professionals who reviewed or otherwise commented on the approach I have taken are: medical doctors Paul Rosenberg, emergency room physician, Toronto, Ontario; Michael Weinstock, family practitioner, Toronto, Ontario; Arthur Waltzer, surgeon, Tampa, Florida; recreation therapist Denise Altschul, Toronto, Ontario; Fredda Vladeck, director, New York Aging in Place Initiative; Robert McMullen, executive director, Abbeyfield Houses Society of Canada; and the property management team of my "vertical village:" Marcie Sherwood, David Colvin, and Judy Creamer. Norman and Judy Barron, who knew my mother and me over a span of decades and understand assisted living facilities, gently provided support and advice to me when it was most needed.

The staff at "Glengrove" (the assisted living facility portrayed in this book and whose name has been fictionalized) shared institutional experiences with me. Some were positive; others, in effect, were "war" stories. I honor their requests (some expressed, others implied) for anonymity. They, too, have fictitious names in the book. They include: "Susan," the residential manager; "Anne," the dining room manager; "Sally," the bank manager; "Cindy," the activities director; "Bee," the apartments' licensed practical nurse; and the volunteers, including "Simon." You know who you are. I thank you.

My mother entered Glengrove close to the age of 90, relatively healthy with a close-knit support system of family, extended family and friends that remained in place until her passing. First among the family was her grandson, my son, Aaron. His was a pervasive, but laid-back presence. Aaron and my mother were frequently on the phone. One of her more ardent wishes was that Aaron would marry. (She wished the same for me, but with the passing years probably gave that hope up as a lost cause.) Aaron did marry, but the event came after my mother's passing. She would have loved my new daughter-in-law, T'mimah (who helped me with the Hebrew part of the dedication to this book).

Even after my brother's death, my mother was included in the warm and loving circle of his widow, Barbara, and her mother, Rita, plus brothers, sisters and children. They gave me further insight into the strength of family in living one's life fully and independently.

Then, there was my mother's immediate family consisting of her nieces and nephews (and some of their children). They were responsive to her (and to me). Several lived close by, such as Mel and Irene, who, on occasion, took emergency calls about my mother from Glengrove. And, on several holidays, they had my mother and her special friend, "Alice," for dinner. Others lived farther away. My cousins Herb and Doris often telephoned. Herb arranged flight tickets for Aunt Lil to visit my mother, and he followed with visits of his own. As well, there were Aunt Dolly; her sons Brandy and Bob; plus my cousins Muriel, Max, Carol, Barbara and Gene; and also my cousins' children Betsy, Lauren and David.

I have fictionalized Glengrove and many of its staff and officers—but what I have written faithfully reflects both my mother's and my understanding that Glengrove was committed to achieving an environment that would foster independent living and aging in place. But, we also came to understand that, as is the case in many assisted living facilities, there were inherent conflicts between aging in place and the capacity for independent living. Fictionalizing Glengrove and its staff and officers has allowed me the freedom to define that conflict.

DANIEL JAY BAUM

Toronto, Ontario, 2007

ASSISTED LIVING

FOR OUR PARENTS

Introduction

Three years ago my mother died in an assisted living facility. Almost seven years earlier, at my suggestion, she left the home where she had lived for over forty years and moved into a one-bedroom apartment in a not-for-profit complex constructed with the help of the local Jewish community. Her stay there went relatively smoothly so long as she remained healthy. But episodes of illness and injury punctuated her stay, and finally she experienced the inevitable decline that led to her death.

Her moving into an assisted living facility (ALF) seemed like the best option for both of us. When my mother became more fragile and less able to cope on her own, we could have sold her house, moved her into an apartment, and hired extra help during the day—a solution that we could have afforded. Or perhaps she could have moved in with me. I was her only living child, and we were close. But I was single and divorced, lived in Canada hundreds of miles away, and had a full life of my own. Having her live with me, or close to me, wasn't practical for either of us. My mother would not have wanted to leave behind her many friends in the city where she had lived all her life, so I doubt that she would have accepted the offer.

Assisted living attracted us by its promise of "aging in place." This would allow my mother to navigate gracefully the passage between independence and dependence. She would live in a place that would respect her adult independence yet recognize her growing need for assistance. She would get help in recreating a community, and she would have some stability and control in her life during her waning years. We would both find security and peace of mind.

The facility did not fulfill its promise, however. While it gave lip service to independence, residents there lost control over major areas of their lives—both physical and financial—long before they lost the capacity to make decisions.

Although my mother's final decline was relatively brief, it left an imprint with which I am still trying to cope. I understand that the strength of my reaction to her death is colored by my grief. However, I have shared my experiences with others whose parents have died in assisted living facilities, and I have come to understand that my mother's experience was neither unique nor just a matter of bad luck. Rather, it was the logical outcome of a new American way of death that seems to be almost built into the ALF experience.

Although plenty of books can guide adult children in caring for aging parents, few deal with the relatively new and increasingly popular phenomenon called the assisted living facility.[1] Indeed, before we made the choice to move my mother into an ALF—and even for several years afterward—I wasn't clear about what distinguishes an assisted living facility from an independent living facility or a skilled nursing home. Now I have grasped at least some of the nuances and the policy reasons behind them. But how many adult children or their parents understand the bargain they make when they sign an open-ended ALF contract? How many know what to look for and what will be delivered when their parents choose to "age in place"? How many make what amounts to an impulse purchase? How many have sufficient knowledge to help their parents cope with the many surprises of assisted living?

I wrote this book to help aging parents and their adult children understand the problems and risks in choosing an ALF, with the hope that they might avoid some of the experiences my mother and I had. My story echoes many other people's stories.

But of course I don't pretend that what I will describe happens to everyone entering an ALF.

My mother was relatively affluent and, with my financial help, could afford a high-end facility, where monthly rents then ranged from $1,700 to $6,000. (I know that most people don't have that luxury.) She also had family members to watch out for her. (For people who have no family, assisted living is often their only option, and one that they have to navigate alone.) My mother also had a zest for life that not all the elderly enjoy. She had not suffered the fate of many women her age—surviving the recent death of a spouse—and so did not view an ALF as merely a place to end her life.

I also know that many people have had more positive experiences than those I will recount, while others have had even more problematic ones. For many who have a will to live while they still "have their wits" about them, as my mother put it, life in an ALF can be exciting and marked by moments of hope and learning, yet it can also be enervating, frustrating, and sometimes frightening.

My mother was typical of the strongest among the two hundred thousand Americans—mostly women—who become residents of assisted living facilities each year. And Glengrove was a typical high-end facility. It was a modern complex of fifty assisted living apartments (one- or two-bedroom units), sixty "suites" (each consisting of one large room partitioned for sitting, eating, and sleeping), and a nursing home with a maximum capacity of 230 beds in either single or shared rooms. For much of my mother's stay, the nursing home, like many such facilities, was significantly underutilized, with only slightly more than half of the beds occupied. The apartment residents referred to the nursing home and its attached skilled care unit as the "sick building"—a place they generally feared because of its association with further loss of freedom, removal from their apartments and, finally, with death.

Though nominally open to all, Glengrove was a combined effort of the city's Jewish community, where economies of scale brought Orthodox, Conservative, and Reform groups together. Compromises of a sort had been made, for example, with regard to dietary laws, keeping Kosher, and traditions like keeping the Sabbath, when, to illustrate, the elevators worked automatically, not on manual button direction. There were two synagogues—one Orthodox and the other Reform, both with young rabbis. A member of the Glengrove board of directors once asked the Jewish community's supervising elderly Orthodox rabbi, "So what will you do if a resident makes a non-kosher meal in her apartment?" With a bit of a twinkle the rabbi answered, "I set rules, but I'm not a policeman."

My mother had a strong hold on life, a sense of humor, and an interest in others in the ALF and in the community outside. If my mother could make a good life for herself in what appeared to be a typical high-end ALF, I was sure others like her might do the same. I wasn't thinking only of my mother's future. I was sixty-three when my mother moved from her home. Although I had long acted to be financially secure, only recently had I begun to think about how I would live my life as the years passed.

I was sure I would be in a good position to monitor and to help my mother. I assumed that my education, training, and work enabled me to be an aware observer and a strong advocate. Observing, asking questions, probing for facts, and sensing emotions had been part of my adult life as a reporter for a major daily newspaper, a graduate student in law, a lawyer and law professor, a labor arbitrator and human rights adjudicator, and a writer on public policy questions.

What I discovered was that I had limited ability to influence my mother's experience. Although I constantly sought information related not only to her experiences but to those of other residents, as well as staff and volunteers, I felt powerless to affect the events that hastened her decline and death. If someone with my skills and education could not help a loved one, what would happen to someone who was less affluent, less assertive, and lacked skill as an advocate?

The not-for-profit assisted living facility where my mother lived was an institution bent on doing good—or at least doing as little harm as possible. In writing this book I describe the pressures that administrators and staff deal with daily. To a considerable extent, however, what I describe reflects my perceptions and those of my mother. Because they may not reflect the intentions of those who ran the ALF, I have changed its name as well as the identities of individuals, and I have not identified the American city where it is located.

In this book I recount my mother's years at Glengrove and my experiences trying to help her live there in a positive way. I evaluate my success or failure in maintaining her quality of life and respecting her wishes. And most important, I examine the assumptions I made—and abandoned—as I helped my mother negotiate life in her new home.

For example, I originally thought I was helping my mother to choose how to live her final years. But on what basis could she choose, and what was my role in effecting that choice? I also assumed that my money would enhance her quality of life, but later I wondered about that.

I was concerned about social isolation. Her quality of life would depend on her sense of security and comfort in her new surroundings. She was a social person and made friends both at Glengrove and outside. She built a deep support system of people among whom there was mutual caring. But could she maintain that community as she became more frail and aged in place? Could an ALF be a place of security? Would she get appropriate medical care that would help her maximize her strengths and cope with her weaknesses? And what about end-of-life decisions? Would the ALF respect her wish to die in place as well as age in place?

Dealing with my mother's final days and then her death was a wrenching event. She and I had never really talked about these matters. One evening when I came to Glengrove to take her out to dinner, she presented me with a check. She said it was money she had saved over several years and that it was to cover the cost of her funeral. She felt that I had done enough to help her. Almost in passing, she mentioned that she didn't want to be kept alive if she were brain dead. She concluded: "I have no intention of dying anytime soon. . . . Let's go to dinner."

I have often wondered what might have happened if, at the start, I had taken a different approach. What if I had helped her purchase another home, one that could have been renovated for safe use (e.g., with no stairs and with railings along the walls)? What if I had hired the necessary help to enable her to stay in her home? Would these actions have resulted in a better lifestyle? Would they have given her continued independence, including the right to die in her own home with dignity?

For my mother, the answer to these questions now have no meaning. She died in the "sick building" at Glengrove. But I hope that what I learned will help other adult children and their parents understand how to take greater personal control of their lives.

What happens to our parents on their final journey affects us, their adult children. One day we will be making the same journey. How we help our parents may shape how we respond when our children, our friends, or other relatives try to help us. One day most of us will make such choices, or they will be made for us. We travel in our parents' wake.

1   Choice

In my mother's eighty-ninth year, it seemed only a matter of weeks before I sensed that she could no longer live safely in her home. The suddenness of that realization came as a shock. For more than forty years, she had lived independently in her small home, a two-bedroom bungalow with a garage, basement, and small yard. My mother did not share my concerns. She was her own person, though with the passing years she looked increasingly to me for advice.

She had always seemed a bundle of energy. Under five feet tall, bright-eyed, intelligent, she preferred to listen before talking. She would bide her time. Then, she would speak her mind. She held strong moral and political views with regard to religion, Israel, and her sense of family. She was a hardened Democrat. Franklin Delano Roosevelt could have done no wrong. Morally, Clinton was flawed ("He's a man, just a man") but was still a good president. Being Jewish was important, especially during the High Holy Days. For a Jew, marrying or even fraternizing outside the Jewish religion was wrong. Whatever the issue, Israel was to be supported. Her family, both immediate and extended, was central to her. She always seemed to be there for me, though for decades she worked a forty-hour week.

My mother came from a modern Orthodox Jewish family of five children (four daughters and a son), seemingly dominated by my grandfather. "Seemingly" in the sense, as my mother told it, that if she or her siblings did any wrong, they could count on my grandmother telling my grandfather and then saying to him in Russian, "Don't spank the children." My mother graduated from high school—no small achievement in those post–World War I days.

My father was a loving person with strong views shaped by the realities of adolescent enlistment and service in the trenches of World War I. He had only a fifth-grade education, and during the Depression of the 1930s he lost his job as a shoe store manager and had to labor as an unskilled factory worker. Like my grandfather, he was master of the house—subject to being overridden, usually quietly, by my mother. My father, like my older brother, was a heavy smoker. They both died of lung cancer after long, painful illnesses during which my mother stayed by their side. She grieved deeply and openly, and then got on with her life.

Caring for her home, keeping it spotless, and making improvements had been a major source of pride for my mother. She had no help, nor did she want any. She scrubbed the floors, painted the walls, and shoveled the snow. When she was ill, her wish was to be left alone. She, nature, and God would see to her cure.

There also were times when fast-talking salespeople had taken advantage of her. There was, for example, the "lawn-improvement" company that had promised a greener, more beautiful yard, which it would service. The chemical mix that they sprayed on the yard turned the grass brown, and the maintenance service never materialized. My mother had seen this merely as a bump along the path of daily life. She was aware that there were predators out there who preyed on the weak and vulnerable. She was aware, too, that some of them would even try to steal her identity. "That's why I don't give my Social Security number to anyone," she said. But she did not think such wrongs could happen to her; her outlook was positive.

My mother had many creative outlets. She was known among

relatives and friends—and indeed throughout her neighbor-hood—as a great baker. Her special holiday packages of strudel were much anticipated. The recipe was her secret, but since I wanted to pass it on to family members, my mother agreed to give it to me, on the condition that the teaching was to be by doing. Everything was to be done from scratch. That meant making the dough, rolling it paper thin, chopping walnuts, sort-ing and filling pastry rolls. The process took hours. I finished in a sweat. Leaning against the kitchen wall, this little woman, who made strudel as a matter of course several times each year, looked at me with a sweet, sad smile and said, "I'm sorry it was so hard for you."

My mother had always worked outside the home. Her first full-time job was as a shoe saleswoman, and her boss (for two years before their marriage) was my father. Later, and for much of her adult life until she was forced to retire at sixty-five, she was a top salesperson (of men's underwear) in the city's leading department store.

My mother had a love of work and didn't want to retire. She enjoyed meeting customers and making sales and felt confident that customers would return. Even toward the end of her life, she would comment on the quality of retail service, sometimes praising and sometimes criticizing, but always intimating that she was still a salesperson at heart. Her forced retirement came when the department store for which she worked changed own-ership and the president, who used to visit and congratulate her on the sales floor, himself was shown the door.

One day while I was in town visiting my mother soon after she retired, my friend Larry and I met and, over a glass of wine, hatched a plan: Why not give my mother the opportunity to profit from her strudel? Let her see the commercial value in it, and maybe she would have the urge to start a new business that we would be happy to help finance.

Larry made a reservation for dinner at Les Arbres, a well-known local restaurant. We then stopped by and left some of my mother's strudel (from a box she had given me) with Armand, the maître d', and put some special plans in place.

That evening, my mother and I joined Larry and his wife, Judy, at Les Arbres. We talked and joked through our appetizers and main courses. Then came dessert. Armand said that he had something special for us: there on an elaborately decorated pastry tray was my mother's strudel. She looked surprised, and then she laughed. Armand, rather seriously, said that it was no laughing matter. He already had sold ten pieces at seven dollars each. If my mother would bake more, he would be pleased to feature her strudel as a special dessert. Without hesitating, my mother thanked Armand but firmly said no. Her strudel was for family and friends. She had left the world of paid work. She owned her home, and she had a small pension and Social Security checks to support her.

My mother was frugal, though it seemed that throughout her life there were always more debts than cash to pay them. Still, she managed to make ends meet. Her only real asset was her modest home for which the mortgage had been paid some five years earlier. Except for home improvements, such as central air conditioning and carpeting, she had continued to spend little and to shop for bargains.

She lived contentedly, and if anyone had told her she was living close to the poverty level, she would have been insulted. She saw herself as independent and middle-class, in no small measure because of the independence that her home provided. Indeed, her home, in her eyes, was an estate that she wanted to pass on to my son, Aaron.

I had worried about my mother in retirement. How would she spend her days? Would she become fixated on television? Would solitude lead to depression? I need not have worried. She often had dinner parties for a dozen or more people—a joy to her and her guests. She prepared at least four courses for these meals and served the food on her unmatched but much-envied end-of-line pieces of china. During the last two years before she moved into Glengrove, my mother relented and allowed some of her guests to help clear the table and wash the dishes. (She had refused the gift of a dishwasher.)

A LIFE CHANGE?

Things changed dramatically about ten months before my mother turned ninety. Until then her world was vibrant and balanced. Even at eighty-nine she took pleasure in traveling by plane from her home to visit me in Toronto, agreeing to the use of a wheelchair in the airport only because she was carrying such a heavy load of strudel.

Yet, in a matter of months death took many of my mother's friends who were important parts of her support system. The death of her family doctor and longtime friend, Walter Gold, saddened her. She had often visited his home and had become a second grandmother to his children. Then she lost her sister, the matriarch of the family. My Aunt Rose was a tiny woman with a great heart and a big car—which she often drove with my mother as a passenger. My mother and Aunt Rose, whose husband had died years before, had been close. And then there was Josephine, her neighbor across the street, who frequently came by for late-night chats. Aunt Rose and Josephine died quickly within weeks of each other.

My mother also witnessed the end of the neighborhood she had known. Her synagogue, which my grandfather had founded, had moved miles away. Aunt Rose used to drive there with my mother; now there was no readily available transportation. So, too, her favorite kosher-style food store posted a notice that it would soon move to a distant location.

My mother's situation—an elderly parent living alone and losing her support system—impelled me to begin some general reading and to converse with similarly situated friends. What I learned from my initial research was perhaps obvious to many people: the experience of changing neighborhoods and worlds is widely shared. It is, of course, the nature of any community to change. For older residents, however, change becomes more pronounced as families move away and friends pass on. They respond by drawing the wagons of their life into ever tighter circles. So long as there is the intimacy of close family ties, basic good health, and the desire to live, positive approaches to aging and to getting on with life—even including death—exist.

But for me the reality was complicated by distance. My mother's home—and that meant her friends, family, and surroundings since birth—was a U.S. city almost a thousand miles away. Mine, for more than thirty-five years, had been Toronto. I telephoned regularly and visited often, but I could not be there on a daily basis to help and, if necessary, monitor her well-being. Of course, some elderly parents do move in with their children, but for my mother, a move to a distant city would have ranked as among the worst of possible alternatives.[1]

What I wanted for my mother was, I believe, what she wanted for herself: her own space, freedom to structure her own use of time, and the ability to care for herself. So long as she remained healthy, there was a good possibility she could remain in her own home. She ate well, preparing healthy food that she enjoyed and continuing to create new recipes. She had designed an at-home exercise program involving the use of a bungee cord. Still, her cholesterol had gone up to worrisome levels. Also, laser surgery to remove cataracts really hadn't seemed to help what was a degenerative condition. Reading, which my mother enjoyed, had been sharply curtailed.

My mother got to the eye surgeon (or, rather, he got to my mother) before I was aware of what he had proposed. She had heard of him through a television solicitation and from some acquaintances. She accepted what she heard. In both his TV advertising and his interview with my mother, he promised that the laser procedure would be painless and effective. He said nothing about the recovery period and, like many patents, she didn't ask. He promised that my mother's already limited sight would be restored to 20/20. What is more, on the day of the procedure, she would be picked up in a limousine and returned home. Medicare and her private insurance would cover the cost.

My mother got the limo ride, no bill, and pain that lasted for several days. The doctor prescribed powerful eye drops that she clearly had difficulty administering and which, several months later, contributed to dizziness, a fall, and a brief hospital stay.

Yet, at the time, what concerned me even more were falls my mother had taken because she continued to climb a short ladder to clean walls and change light bulbs. When she fell, she assured me that the only result was "a bruise." But this led me to think about the steep stairs to her basement where she did her laundry. A fall there might be the end. My mother laughed it off. I didn't. I was aware that the largest number of deaths for those over sixty-five in the United States and Canada are the result of falls.[2] (Falls often may signal underlying physical problems.)

If a fall weren't the end, it could be the start of a path to dependence. Age had not limited my mother's ability to get around. But if she was confined to a wheelchair or, worse, to a bed, her life would change dramatically. At the very least, she would be dependent on others. It might not be impossible for her to get about, but it would be difficult for someone who so valued her independence.

My concern about my mother increased when I read of people who had lived, apparently in good health, into their late eighties and then suddenly took tumbles. Sometimes medical alert systems were in place but the injured persons could not send a signal for help. People were sometimes left alone in their homes or gardens until someone—by accident—found them after hours or even days. I did not want that to happen to my mother.

I asked myself if I might be acting on my fears and concerns, and not in her best interest. After all, she still had the run of her own home. But there were danger signs, such as tripping on the living room rug and a recent fall while standing on a ladder. And I could not get those steep basement steps out of my mind.

I thought it might be possible to lessen these dangers by seeking the advice of an expert.

PREVENTIVE ACTION SUGGESTED AND REFUSED

I talked to my mother's doctor and made a tentative appointment to have a geriatric nurse visit her to discuss how to make her home safer. Geriatric nursing assessments, if acted on, often allow elderly parents to continue to live in their own homes. As the doctor cautioned, however, both parents and adult children need to decide how to respond when a troubling incident signals incipient incapacity.

After explaining carefully what the nurse would do, I assured my mother that the nurse would be making suggestions that could be accepted or rejected. When I hung up the phone, I thought I had my mother's approval. But the nurse told me that when she phoned to make an appointment, my mother refused. This was her home, my mother said. She didn't need to have anyone going through it suggesting changes. She might have had falls, but none was serious enough to force her to bed or to a hospital. Leave well enough alone.

My mother remained firm in her view. I will never know whether she could have stayed longer in her home if the nurse had made a safety assessment and it had guided our actions.

MY ROLE: CROSSING THE LINE—FROM ADVICE TO ACTION

My mother's refusal to get the advice of a geriatric nurse brought to a head many of my concerns regarding her well-being. She wanted to stay in her own home—and I wanted what was important to her. I believed, however, that she might need help. But my mother, who was mentally alert and certainly had no problems making decisions, refused help. This is a typical scenario and one that illuminates a central difficulty of independent living. My mother was her own person. She might act in a way that risked her health and even her life, but what right did I have to challenge such action? And even if she accepted help now, that assistance might not suffice for tomorrow. The geriatric nurse had reminded me that our needs change as we grow older.

I found myself raising critical questions with my mother: Was her home becoming a burden? Was there value in looking at alternatives such as assisted living facilities?

I didn't know much about assisted living facilities when I first made this suggestion. I couldn't have explained the differences among an "assisted living facility," an "independent living facility," and a "continuing care community." I still can't—nor, it seems, can many of the experts. When I checked definitions online while writing this book, the website of the American Association of Retired Persons (AARP) reported that states have "varying definitions" of what actually constitutes an assisted living facility.[3]

According to the AARP website, ALFs differ in their philosophies and their management style, and in how they deal with the issue of residents' independence and privacy: "The lack of agreement on a definition makes it difficult to obtain consistent data on assistive living."

Because AARP had trouble collecting consistent data, I relied on what I could research, along with the advertising of facilities near my mother. They all assured me that she could have her own apartment, meals, entertainment, and help for any medical emergencies.

I had crossed an important line. No longer was I simply offering to help my mother with minor matters while gently raising questions and advice for her to accept or reject concerning her lifestyle. I had moved beyond completing her tax returns (usually with the help of my friend Larry's wife, Judy) and dealing sometimes with dubious bills from merchants. I was now an advocate trying to persuade my mother to make a decision about a choice that I had reached: She should leave her home for a different lifestyle, with economic security bottomed on my resources rather than hers.

The proceeds from the sale of her home would be used to pay her rent at the ALF, but the income and capital would sustain her for less than three years. After that time, I would handle rent, medical services not otherwise covered by Medicare, and supplemental insurance, as well as the cost of prescription drugs. This was a responsibility that I willingly assumed. But it was also a responsibility, I now understood, that any assisted living facility contractually imposes.

I am not sure of all that went through my mother's mind and heart when she was faced with my questions and arguments. All that she said was that she understood she was getting old and that she couldn't stay in her home forever. Then it seemed that—quietly and without expressly saying so—she accepted the decision to move from her home to an ALF. She acted on my judgment. After all, where were the data that would allow her— or me, for that matter—to determine the comparable worth of different institutions and then assess that data in relation to continued life at home? In any event, I believe it was emotion, not objective criteria, that guided my mother. She felt vulnerable, and she trusted me. In a factual sense the decision to move was hers. In a more fundamental sense, the decision was mine. There is little doubt in my mind that my mother understood that she had passed this decision to me, as well as the ongoing responsibility that came with it.

I was not happy about what I had done. I had encouraged my mother, and she had agreed to give up an important measure of her independence, namely, control over her money, her home, and her security. I knew that my actions were the same as those of many adult children. As a number of my friends put it, they had begun to parent their parents.

Yet, I did not want to parent my mother. I simply wanted her to be more secure and free to decide what she wanted. I understood, however, that there might well be points along the way when I would have to intercede, either because she wouldn't be able to act on her own behalf or because her decisions wouldn't serve her real interests. In so doing, I was not only making a one-time decision but also assuming ongoing responsibility that would require many decisions in the coming years.

There is little doubt that I had taken something valuable from my mother—an important means to assert her independence. Ultimately, I would be using my money to provide for her. Indeed, there were few financial matters that would be left in her control. Her home would be sold, and her limited pension and Social Security checks would do no more than buy her some outings to the grocery or department store or to a show. I was aware that there were professionals, such as Donna Wagner, a gerontologist and director of the Center for Productive Aging at Towson University in Maryland, who, to say the least, would have frowned on my decision. As Wagner categorically explained: "After losing power over so many domains of your life, this is a message that you've gone beyond the age of maturity and we're [the adult children] going to take over. . . . It's insulting."[4]

Nonetheless, I believed my actions were necessary to serve my mother's interests. I would try to find ways to ensure she would retain the maximum amount of freedom. Yet, on reflection several years later, I question whether other choices more sensitive to my mother's independence might not have served both of us better.

RESIDENT PROFILE

When "we" made the decision to find an assisted living facility, my mother seemed to fit the resident profile of those two hundred thousand Americans moving into ALFs in 2000. That year, 70 percent of them left their own homes and funded their stay in the ALFs largely from the sale of those homes. As one major study of ALFs—the *High Service High Privacy Study,* published in 2000—explained: "The residents in the high privacy or high service ALFs were largely white, widowed females, who were quite elderly. More than one-half of the residents were 85 years of age or older."[5] These residents entered ALFs where the rent was about what my mother would be paying: $1,700 per month. Most were relatively well educated and had moved into an ALF from their own home or apartment. Interestingly, the study noted that the decision to enter some sort of independent living facility was not usually made independently. The vast majority of those studied had help—almost always from adult children. One-quarter of residents indicated that they had "little or no control over the decision to enter a facility."[6]

HOME SOLD, ALF SELECTED

Many decisions had to be made before my mother moved. Her home had to be sold, which meant that I had to find and deal with a real estate agent who would be hundreds of miles from where I lived. I spoke with friends familiar with my mother's neighborhood and with real estate agents who had handled a number of sales there. I found an agent who was himself elderly, had worked with elderly sellers, and seemed like a patient person. We set up a three-way line of communication among my mother, the agent, and myself. We had to make decisions with regard to posting a For Sale sign, arranging for house inspections, and reviewing possible offers.

I felt it important for my mother to understand the value of her home, which was determined by looking at the recent sale prices of comparable homes in her neighborhood. Over a period of weeks, she got into the sale mode. She wanted to be present when the agent brought viewers to inspect her house, and to answer their questions. This was her home and she was proud of it. She had questions of her own concerning the final offer. When they were answered, she approved of the buyer—a single mother purchasing her first home.

The buyer barely had money for a down payment. Financing

was difficult but it was obtained with a first and second mortgage. It was my mother's idea to sell to the buyer many of her
furnishings—in particular, those of the second bedroom and
dining room—at a low price. She decided to give her the rest,
except for what she would need for her new home. "I'm not
going to get much for this, and it will give her a chance to have
a fully furnished home. She has enough expenses already."

There was a kind of momentum and excitement connected
with the sale of the home. Yet, I wondered whether my mother
grasped what the sale actually meant. After all, she was continuing to live in her home just as she had done for more than forty
years. Would the reality of leaving her home forever come when
she walked out the door for the last time?

In the meantime, one of my mother's first questions was
whether there would be sufficient time to find an ALF and to
furnish her new home before closing on her old one. We had
about two months, and she seemed satisfied. I wasn't so sure.

My focus in evaluating an ALF centered on its physical layout
and the services it offered, such as handling medical emergencies. My mother's central concern, however, seemed to be location in an area with a large Jewish population, as well as one
with shops and markets where she would feel comfortable.

There were two high-end facilities that seemed to meet my
mother's criteria. One was a for-profit ALF that had operated
for several years. It had a relatively large Jewish population, but
it had no Jewish cultural program. It had no rabbi or minister of
any faith on site. Though the rents were high, the apartments
did not seem spacious. But it was located close to places where
my mother liked to shop.

The fact that it was a for-profit institution concerned me. I
didn't know whether the institution's focus on profit would always square with a commitment to the welfare of its residents.

Much of the ownership of assisted living facilities—which
number in the thousands of "beds," as residents usually are cat-
egorized—is in the hands of for-profit corporations, whose

stocks often are listed on exchanges. Consider these 1999 assisted living for-profit corporation figures: Alterra Health Care Corporation, based in Milwaukee, Wisconsin, had 20,653 beds in 450 facilities; Emeritus Assisted Living, in Seattle, Washington, had 13,400 beds in 130 facilities; Marriott Senior Living Services, in Washington, DC, had 11,603 beds in 144 facilities; and Sunrise Assisted Living, in McLean, Virginia, had 10,906 beds in 140 facilities. The top thirty U.S. assisted living companies in 1999 increased their resident capacity by 24 percent over that of 1998, from 127,101 beds to 157,249 beds in the hands of for-profit chains.[7]

I was also worried that a for-profit ALF might seem stable and attractive but would actually be subject to the vagaries of the market. From a study I did and book I wrote several decades ago about Canadian nursing homes, I knew that corporate imperatives to maximize profits often conflict with residents' need for stability.[8] When a number of the nursing homes I studied closed and residents were moved to other locations, there was a significant spike in the patient mortality rate.

Volatility is as true of ALFs as of nursing homes. While I was researching the for-profit versus not-for-profit issue, I found that in 1998 Marriott actually decreased its capacity by two thousand beds. Sunrise Assisted Living nearly doubled its size at the end of 1998 when it acquired twenty-eight facilities from Toledo-based Manor Care.

If labor costs increased and began to eat into profits, then the enterprise might well decide to cut staff to save money, change the population mix in the facility, or increase rent—sometimes far in excess of the amount the resident initially paid. In some facilities, tenants may find themselves in an entirely different population mix if the ALF is unable to maintain high occupancy. In order to assure high occupancy, some ALFs designed for healthier seniors were accepting residents who would otherwise go into nursing homes because they were no longer able to function independently. Sunrise Assisted Living, a for-profit enterprise, at one point told its investors that for some of its facilities it was marketing to "the frailest of the frail."[9]

Residents may also face skyrocketing rents. Of course, rents can increase in both for-profit and not-for-profit organizations. The bottom line exerts pressure on both types of institution, though the need for profits to satisfy investors, it seemed to me at the time, imposed a special pressure on for-profit institutions. For residents, the result of increased rents often is the same: their savings, used for ALF expenses such as rent, become exhausted and they have to turn to their children for support. But when that support is not available, they become merely residents unable to pay their rent. That means that if the adult child who signed as guarantor cannot or will not pay, the resident is out, and the adult child who signed as guarantor assumes care. Consider the following story about what happened to a resident of a for-profit institution:

Keith Stauffer, a retired U.S. Secret Service Agent, placed his mother, eighty-seven, in Sunrise Assisted Living, a for-profit ALF, in Bluemont Park, Arlington, Virginia. Stauffer's mother, who had memory loss but was physically healthy, had savings of $100,000. After fully disclosing his mother's savings, Stauffer asked the facility's marketing director what would happen after those savings were exhausted. He was told not to worry. The ALF would seek some small payments from the family, and Medicaid would take care of the rest. The director's promise was not part of the lengthy contract Stauffer and his mother had signed.

Four years later, Stauffer's mother was still alive but her savings were gone. The marketing director no longer was employed by the ALF. Bills for ALF rent and services quickly mounted. Stauffer's mother (and Stauffer) owed $20,000. The ALF director did not deny the representations claimed to be made by the former marketing director. But those representations had not been made part of the contract of tenancy. The director said that he would have to discharge her.

One night in January 2001, Stauffer took his mother out for dinner and never brought her back to the ALF. He had found a nursing home that would take her and accept payment from Medicaid for her stay.[10]

There are also for-profit ALFs that, in order to attract customers with limited means, initially discount rates which they will later increase. From the ALF's point of view, such tenants are a way of filling unused space. At a later point, once the tenant is part of the ALF community, the guarantor family will be under considerable personal pressure to find additional funds for increased rent.

In the only national study of former assisted-living residents, fewer than one in ten people reported leaving because they had run out of money. Yet, nearly one-third of assisted-living residents discovered they needed to pay more than they had expected.[11]

In the event of higher rents, what choice would a resident without a guarantor with additional assets have but to stretch a probably already tight budget and pay the increase? Once a person moves into an ALF, it is no easy matter for her to uproot herself and move out. In my mother's case, I was able to handle the ALF's expenses, although by the end of her stay the cost stretched my resources.

A chief reason that costs or other changes cannot always be foreseen was suggested in a federal examination of the industry's marketing practices in the United States. In 1999 the General Accounting Office, the investigative arm of the U.S. Congress, conducted a study of assisted living. According to the analysis of facilities in four states, only one facility in four gives prospective customers a copy of its contract before they decide to move in.[12]

Once new residents are given contracts, the documents can be "vague or really complicated," said Stephanie Edelstein, who studied ALFs as an attorney for the American Bar Association's Commission on Legal Problems of the Elderly. For example, a contract might say that a facility provides meals, without spelling out that the basic rate includes two meals a day, leaving residents to pay extra for a third meal and snacks.

Similarly, when AARP recently surveyed dozens of facilities in eight states, it found that marketing brochures frequently promise more services than the contracts guarantee. In the advertising world, this might be called "puffing." The Federal Trade Commission might consider such statements as deceptive advertising.

On balance, it seemed to me that there were more risks for my mother with a for-profit corporation than a not-for-profit. A nonprofit's goal, at least on paper, generally is to enhance the quality of life of its residents, allowing them to the extent possible to age in place. Profit is not a central goal. Obviously, a not-for-profit operates on a budget reflecting revenues from contributions and resident rents. Surely, there are occasions when a nonprofit's budget is squeezed. I assumed, however, that the administration of a not-for-profit facility would be focused on the well-being of its residents. And in the final analysis, if budgetary constraints became too burdensome, there was always recourse to the community that had established the ALF.

The other ALF that my mother and I viewed was not-for-profit, newly constructed, and due to open in a few months. Called Glengrove and located in a then-rural setting, close to where many in the Jewish community seemed to be moving, it was an amalgam of two homes for the aged operated by the Orthodox, Conservative, and Reform parts of the city's Jewish community. On one side, there was a large forested area. The buildings, which were attached, covered what seemed to be more than a city block. The ALF portion was a three-story building with about sixty apartments, mostly one-bedroom but with some two-bedroom units. There was a lobby with a fireplace and a piano. On the first floor there was an intimate dining room for the ALF tenants. On the second floor there was an exercise room and a library with computers. A long corridor on the first floor led to the synagogues, cultural center, deli, gift store, health care area, and a nursing home with its skilled nursing unit.

At the time, the area surrounding Glengrove held a rural farming population, from which the management of the facility apparently hoped to draw a part of its labor force. It was their hope that recruits from farming families would be sensitive and committed to the care of the elderly.

As we later discovered, the management was wrong. For the most part, these so-called farming families were more interested in higher-paying jobs available in the city. Glengrove management had to compete for the same labor force as other ALFs— except that competition was more difficult because public transportation to Glengrove was limited.

Careful planning over a period of years went into the design of the buildings, staff policy, its program for aging in place, its sense of Jewish culture, and, not least, a financial base to actualize its program. Management, dedicated volunteers, and directors traveled North America visiting other not-for-profit ALFs. They wanted to do this right; they wanted the best. At least this is what I perceived, and it seemed to be confirmed by two old friends, both of whom had served on Glengrove's board of directors and, before that, on the boards of directors of the Jewish Orthodox Home for the Aged and the Reform Jewish Home.

The admission interview was with the manager of the apartment complex, Susan, a social worker who had long worked for the Reform home. It was clear to me that she was making a quick and subtle assessment of whether my mother would indeed be able to function independently at Glengrove. She listened carefully to my mother and encouraged discussion.

Next there was a tour of the complex, which probably also satisfied any concern Susan might have had as to my mother's ability to walk and her capacity to express herself, as well as her interest in a well-kept home. Adjacent to Susan's office were two other rooms: one for the recreation director and the other for a licensed practical nurse. Each apartment had an emergency cord in every room. Pull the cord, and help would come. It was a kind of local medical alert. That satisfied me. I assumed that nurses and doctors were in the vicinity and would respond.

What my mother saw was quite different. She wanted a second-floor apartment. "You never know who might want to break in. They would have a lot more trouble on the second floor." At the time, inwardly, I laughed at this. After all, there was an office on the main floor. I thought that surely someone would be on duty during the evening hours. I found later that I was wrong. Only after residents and their families complained did the facility hire someone to be on duty at night in the ALF.

My mother asked for permission to return the next day "to take measurements" with her young friend, Lynn. Susan agreed. My mother found that the space would permit her to take all her living room furniture to the one-bedroom apartment. The bedroom and the bathroom were larger than those in her home. There was no bathtub, only a shower stall with a stool. She would miss the tub, but she accepted the explanation that it had been eliminated to prevent falls.

The kitchen was small, and there was no dining room. Still, there was enough space to cook and bake, and she could put a small table in a corner of the living room for meals by herself or with a guest. And there was a dishwasher, which my mother insisted she would never use. She hadn't had one before, and she certainly wasn't going to use one now. After she moved in, however, a friend showed her how to work the dishwasher and she began to use it.

Two meals, lunch and dinner, were served each day within a given time frame. The meals were prepared in the kitchen located in the nursing home section of Glengrove. They were brought by hot carts to the apartment complex. We were assured that the chef wanted to hear from the residents as to the quality of the meals. (This became a joke because new chefs seemed to appear with some frequency.) My mother said that if she didn't like a meal, then she would leave and fix one she did like in her apartment.

There seemed to be a community in which mother could feel comfortable. We walked to the small synagogues—both Orthodox and Reform—on the premises. She liked the idea of a rabbi who would be available.

My mother even knew some of the residents. Some had been neighbors on the street where she lived. The volunteers working in the gift shop and the deli seemed warm and outgoing, and they were there on a regular basis, often for several hours at a time. At one point, several years before, my mother and Aunt Rose often had gone as volunteers to the Orthodox home and served coffee and tea.

Regularly employed bus drivers took residents shopping or on outings, either in a minibus or one of school-bus size. One of the most popular outings was to a riverboat gambling casino, where the buffet was good and inexpensive (five dollars), and the slots took quarters. The minibus was available, at a charge, to take residents to medical appointments.

A few times each week a physical therapist came to the second-floor exercise room to help individual residents set up and carry out an exercise program. The room was open to all those who had a doctor's note certifying that they were healthy enough to work out. My mother obtained a note on her third day at Glengrove. By the fifth day, she had a sweat suit and was in the exercise room.

At the interview with the residence manager, I was presented with a pamphlet titled *Glengrove Apartment Handbook* and a thirteen-page "Resident Agreement." The latter, a legally binding contract, was written simply but with the sure hand of a lawyer intent on a binding agreement with minimal liability to Glengrove.

I must say that I was far more concerned with what the manager and my friends on the Glengrove board said or implied about the place than with what the contract specified. Although I am a lawyer who is used to deciphering contracts, I later learned that I was not very different from many adult children acting for their parents in choosing an ALF. Many of these adult children never received a contract at the time of admission of their parents. They, like me, entered a contract without really understanding—and certainly not questioning—the terms. If a contract were provided before admission, the terms would be set out in print to accept or reject. Only the blanks to accommodate names and dates would be left to be filled in by the residence manager or marketing director. The most that those of us who signed a contract could hope for would be explanations about the meaning of its provisions. And those interpretations seldom were ever included in the written contract.

What was significant to me were the repeated verbal assurances by senior management, almost like a mantra, of an institutional commitment to allow residents to "age in place." To me, this meant that residents who became increasingly frail would be able to remain in their apartments so long as they were not a danger to themselves or to others. They could remain there until death. If additional nursing help were needed, then it would be my responsibility to find and pay for such help. Again, I would discover how wrong I was.

In the admission interview, I did not ask, nor did anyone explain, what would happen as my mother grew increasingly frail. On reflection, I assumed—and I think my mother did as well—that she had several more years of active life if she took proper care of herself. I even hoped that death, rather than senility, would come quickly, perhaps in her sleep. Neither of us envisioned any heightened loss of short-term memory. My mother thought her memory was excellent. She frequently quoted Aunt Rose saying to her, "You would remember where a pin dropped a week after it happened." She had trouble seeing, but with glasses she could still read a newspaper. And though she saw many residents at Glengrove with walkers, they were not for her. She enjoyed long walks. There was no reason they shouldn't continue.

Frankly, I'm not sure that either my mother or I would have welcomed any discussion of what would happen if she grew more frail. Nor do I know if we would have paid greater attention if the residence manager had outlined Glengrove's policy identifying how the facility would handle patients who posed a health risk to themselves.

Would we have listened if they had told us what would happen if my mother's blood pressure rose but she refused to take her medication and adjust her diet? If this was a risk the resident was willing to take, would the ALF leave her alone or would management intervene and monitor her diet? The only mention of risk in the contract, as it turned out, related to smoking. Glengrove was a smoke-free environment. Smoking areas were provided, however, and residents could smoke in their apartments so long as they didn't pose a fire risk.

I know that we didn't want to hear about the details. But perhaps we would have paid greater attention if those details had been carefully and sensitively explained to us. I can't be sure, but I do know that someone should have tried. It would have made the future more understandable.

After my mother and I were interviewed and the basic monthly financial obligations were explained, we were shown the facility and the available apartments. My mother didn't rush to take an apartment. She thought about it, took measurements, shopped for and found a small dining table, and then decided: she would move to Glengrove.

Subtly and not so subtly, I had encouraged and pushed for a life-changing decision that my mother accepted. I soon became aware, as I said before but I will repeat, I wasn't making a one-time decision but was assuming responsibility for choices in the years to come.

2 Moving Day

It was moving day. Weeks ago my mother had planted flowers, just as she had done in years past. They were in bloom. "The new owner might like a garden," she said. Hours before, the movers had come and, quickly and efficiently, boxed all that was to be taken to the apartment at Glengrove.

There were still some things that my mother wanted to give away. She no longer needed her special china for her dinner parties. At Glengrove, her apartment was too small for large gatherings. The little table in the corner of her new living room would allow seating for only a few.

While my mother would not be able to pass on her home to her grandson, Aaron, she could at least give him her china. She knew he loved food. He might have dinner parties and think of her when the table was set and people ate off her china. Aaron was delighted with the gift and promptly had the china packaged and sent off to his home.

Aaron, a long-time resident of Los Angeles, operates a gourmet food manufacturing company. He came to support his grandmother (and me). He is gentle, soft-spoken, and intelligent, and during his stay he frequently held his grandmother's hand. "It makes her feel good, Dad. You should try it."

We sat in my mother's living room for the last time. Her expression was not one of eager anticipation but of fear, sadness, and resignation. "I'm really not sure that I want to make the

move. This has been my home for so long. I love it. But I know
I'm getting older. . . . I'll go." Though visibly shaken, she was
going ahead. I had arranged for rooms at a hotel near Glengrove
so that the next day, after breakfast and a drive around the area,
we could go to the apartment. All of this left me with the nag-
ging question, Was I doing the right thing in moving my mother
to Glengrove?

I had arranged for the assistance of the Helpers, a group of
four middle-aged women whose part-time business was setting
up apartments at various ALFs. Susan, the Glengrove residence
manager, had recommended them. The Helpers reminded me of
an ad for an upscale ALF in Toronto which concludes with a
folksy "We'll even help you move."

Sarah, who spoke for them, said, "We'll meet with your
mother. She can tell us what she wants and we'll do it, just as she
instructs. She won't have to do a thing—just walk into her new,
furnished home. We'll even bake a cake! The smell alone usually
delights the new resident. And there will be fresh flowers."

The Helpers met with my mother at her home before the
move. They had drafted a floor plan for her to fill in, indicating
where she wanted her furniture to be placed. They even recommended a moving company with which, I later learned, they had
a "working relationship."

The move was timed to the hour for pickup, overnight stor-
age, and delivery the next day to Glengrove. The Helpers would
do the unpacking, wash dishes, dust everything, and put the
apartment together as my mother wanted. Although I thought
this would make my mother less anxious, what I should have realized was that by employing the Helpers I also experienced less
stress.

The pickup crew from the movers arrived. In less than an
hour, everything had been loaded onto the moving truck. We
left the house, Aaron holding my mother's hand. I was the last
out the door. A neighbor said good-bye and wished my mother
well. She simply nodded.

We took a long drive around the city, visiting a few parks and talking about Aaron's life. In passing, Aaron and I spoke of how exciting my mother's new life was going to be. My mother said little. Then we went to the hotel where the three of us would spend the night, and we had dinner. We continued to chat, though my mother said nothing more about her sadness or regret. But the sense I had was that those feelings continued to weigh on her.

In the morning, before Aaron appeared for breakfast, I met my mother in the lobby. She was smiling and said that she was determined to make her new home work out. She told me of a dream she had the previous night: her husband, my father, had appeared and told her that he wanted her to have a happy life in the apartment, and she had promised to try. There was a kind of lift to her voice when she told me this, and she asked if I thought she was silly for believing in ghosts. I said no. And that was true. My father's presence was real to her.

After breakfast, my mother said that she didn't want to drive around. She wanted to go to her apartment and check on the unpacking. It was clear that she was not about to leave "setting up" the apartment to the Helpers. This was her new home, and she intended to take full possession of it. Nobody needed to bake a cake for her. She could do that herself. Nor did she want any cut flowers. "They die too quickly."

When we arrived at Glengrove, nine residents—seven women and two men—were at the entrance. Some were sitting on benches, some in wheelchairs, and others with walkers beside them. They were watching flowers being planted. Some of the gardeners chatted with them, but none asked the residents for advice, let alone to join in.

This puzzled me because Glengrove had a website that prominently featured its certification as an Eden Alternative facility. The Eden Alternative Movement—sometimes called "Eldertopia"—was founded by William H. Thomas, a physician, who explained his vision:

I want an alternative to the institution. The best alternative I can
think of is a garden. I believe when we make a place that's worthy of
our elders, we make a place that enriches all of our lives—caregivers,
family members, and elders alike. So the Eden Alternative provides a
reinterpretation of the environment elders live in, going from an institution to a garden. That's why we call it the Eden Alternative.

I want people to ask themselves, "What kind of place is this?"
There are kids running around and playing. There are dogs and cats
and birds, and there are gardens and plants. I want people to think
that this can't be a nursing home. Which it isn't—it's an alternative to
a nursing home.[1]

Among other things, this seemed to mean resident participation in creating and caring for gardens that were to form an essential part of their environment. In Ontario, I recalled, a regional
administrator for homes for the aged made a point of having residents help in the planning, planting, and care of gardens.[2]

The residents on the benches didn't simply look at us as we
entered, they stared. My mother responded with a smile. Only a
few returned the gesture. The front office was next to the entrance. Susan was on the phone, but she waved. Bee, a large
African American known as "the nurse," was at her station next
to Susan's office. She smiled broadly and said, "Hello!" I assumed at first that Bee was a registered nurse, but later learned
that she was a licensed practical nurse.

I gave Bee my mother's living will, which included the do-not-
resuscitate provision that she long ago had insisted upon. Bee
glanced at it, said that it seemed to be in order, and assured me
that it would be made a part of my mother's records.

We passed through the warm, somewhat ornate lobby with
its baby grand piano. Five signed Chagall prints donated by the
Friends of Glengrove hung on the walls. There was a large bulletin board which featured a list of the day's activities: yoga, a
Yiddish class, crafts (clay modeling), a chat with the local li-
brarian, and, in the evening, bingo, sponsored by volunteers at
Glengrove.

We took an elevator to my mother's second-floor apartment. The Helpers answered the door. They were surprised to see us and said that they had another few hours of work. Wouldn't we like to come back later? "No," answered my mother. She wanted, where possible, to set up the apartment herself, with the help of her son and grandson.

To the apparent chagrin of the Helpers, my mother told them to forget the cake and flowers. At her direction, Aaron and I moved some furniture and, most important, we hung a group of more than twenty family pictures on the wall leading to the bedroom. This was her "family album." The living room itself was arranged just as it had been in my mother's home. It featured large family photos and also a painting of Aaron done by his mother (Harriet, my ex-wife) and treasured by his grandmother. Now the apartment was as she wanted—at least for the time being.

Lynn, a friend, came with a present which she wasn't sure my mother would accept or use: an answering machine. "My guess is," Lynn said, "that you won't be in the apartment much except to have breakfast and sleep. So people who want to talk with you will have some trouble getting through. They can leave messages, and all you have to do is push the button when you see the red light flashing, wait for the tape to wind, and then listen." To the surprise of Lynn, Aaron, and myself, my mother did indeed think this was a good idea, and she used the machine for several years.

As we worked, visitors arrived, one at a time. Ira, a resident in his seventies, a dignified, well-spoken person, "just wanted to say hello." He asked if my mother would take part in a choir for the dedication of Glengrove upon its final completion the next month. She hesitated, then said "Yes." Ira, who had moved in several months earlier, had been one of Glengrove's first residents.

On his heels came Alice, a bumptious, heavyset woman in her eighties who almost exploded into the apartment. "I'm your next-door neighbor." On the face of it, my mother and Alice seemed so different. Alice was vocal and assertive. Her words seemed to spill out in advance of her thoughts. My mother, for the most part, was restrained, reflective. Yet almost instantly there was a rapport between the two. They were a kind of odd couple. It also seemed as though whatever hesitancy my mother might have had about leaving her home vanished the moment Alice appeared.

They chatted for a while, or rather, Alice spoke and my mother listened. Alice noticed that Aaron and I were there, but she didn't really care; her attention was riveted on her new neighbor. She immediately drew conclusions about my mother: "It's good to have someone here who thinks and is alive. So many of the others only sleep and eat. You'll see. I'll talk with Anne, the dining room manager, and see that we share the same table for meals. I like what you've done with your apartment, but let me show you mine." Alice reached for my mother's arm to shepherd her out the door. My mother smiled, released her arm, and said, "Later, perhaps."

Alice left, but she announced that we would all sit together for dinner. And she emphasized that we had better be there between 5:00 and 5:15 p.m. "because those simply are the hours for serving."

Susan arrived at the apartment next. She just wanted "to see how things were going" and to welcome my mother. She, like Bee—and, for that matter, the entire Glengrove staff—referred to residents by their first names. Initially, my mother noticed and seemed to object. In her view, a person shouldn't be called by her first name unless permission had been granted. Still, in a quiet aside to me, she said: "You know, you have to go along to get along."

This aside told me that my mother recognized a fundamental fact about her new home: she was not taking up residence in an apartment building or in a hotel. If she were a tenant or a hotel guest, there would be clear rights on her side. Without her invitation, no one could invade her privacy. She could come and go as she pleased. She would choose what she ate. Her tenancy would be defined, including its cost which, during the period of lease, could not be increased.

Rather, my mother seemed to understand that she was taking up residence in an institution that had its own rules, enforced by its employees. It was the institution, and those who controlled it, that would now influence the structure of her life. Glengrove might pay homage to the best interests of the residents; yet it would be the institution and not the residents that defined those best interests.

Susan handed my mother two pamphlets that she had given us earlier, the apartment handbook and a glossy four-page advertisement that had been published in the Jewish community's newspaper. My mother glanced at the material. "I am where I am," she said. "The pamphlets are only paper."

My mother asked what I thought she should wear for dinner. She wanted to look nice. I turned to the *Apartment Handbook* and, sure enough, there was a section called "Dress Code," which stated: "Appropriate attire must be worn in public areas at all times—no bathrobes or sleepwear. Gentlemen are requested to wear nice sport clothes at evening meals." This left a large area of decision making for my mother. She wore a bright but not extravagant dress, a simple necklace, and a big smile of anticipation.

My mother was right. The pamphlets were only paper; they were not legal documents. Still, I read them carefully as my mother took her first shower in the apartment and prepared for dinner. For the most part, the pamphlets set out the services included in the room charges.

My mother's room rate for the "first" or basic level of services was $1,700 a month. This provided her with the following:

- two "executive chef" meals (lunch and dinner), served daily in the Glengrove dining room;

- all utilities except telephone;
- light housekeeping (dusting and vacuuming);
- on-site security;
- emergency call service in each room;
- weekly linen service (that is, the washing and drying of linens provided by residents);
- washers and dryers on each floor for resident use;
- "supportive assistance" (which seemed to mean help getting on and off Glengrove's bus);
- a "full, personally tailored activity program" (which seemed to mean freedom for residents to opt into any scheduled program);
- amenities such as a fitness room, beauty and gift shops, and what was called a "neighborhood" deli (because it was located in a common area of the facility);
- access to the health care center (with a doctor's note of permission);
- bus transportation for a per-mile fee; and
- religious services.

I laughed. This was a great time for me to finally pay attention to the details of what we would be paying for at Glengrove. After all, I was the person who had signed a contract of tenancy for my mother, yet I hadn't really read it carefully. However, I was reminded of what my cousin Mel had said of ALFs: Assuming a basic level of care, what really is important to the residents is socializing, being in the company of others. Still, I think I also understood that I had a responsibility to monitor and protect my mother's well-being. I was her advocate.

DINNER AT GLENGROVE

We entered the dining room, navigating around a number of wheelchairs and walkers. This was the domain of Anne, the dining room manager, a solid-looking, no-nonsense person probably in her sixties. Anne had worked in this capacity for more than twenty years at the Orthodox home before it was folded into Glengrove. She was keenly aware of just how important and sensitive the matter of food is to the residents: "It's probably the only subject that will really get them going. Sometimes it doesn't matter if the food is good. Many will always find a reason for fault. That goes with the territory. We listen and try to do the best we can. But this isn't a Hilton."

The job had some frustration for Anne, in no small part because the food was prepared in the kitchens at the other end of Glengrove, near the nursing home quarters. It was brought to the ALF dining room in warmers. So, more often than not, food that should have been hot tended to range from warm to cold. And since the chef was not immediately available, Anne was generally the target for residents' complaints. Still, though she was tough, she could display softness, and she obviously cared about the residents.

Anne greeted my mother warmly and said that she could sit with Alice but had the option of moving to another table in the future. I wasn't sure whether she was delivering a message concerning Alice as a companion. Anne welcomed Aaron and me as guests, who were required to pay a modest fee of five dollars for dinner. (The charge was added to my mother's monthly bill, which was forwarded to me.) "Meals, especially dinners," she said, "are always a pressure cooker." As we walked to the assigned table, several of the faces that had stared at us from benches at the entrance now greeted my mother with a hello. She was now one of them.

Anne said that many of the residents actually came to their tables up to a half hour before meals were served. The dining room was pleasant. It met Glengrove's description of being "intimate." There was no cafeteria decor. Tables were for four or six, and each was covered with fresh linen, china settings, and attractive cutlery. The walls had textured paper and were hung with bright pictures. Vases of flowers dotted the room.

The ambiance, however, was anything but tranquil. There

was a frenetic quality and quite a high level of noise. Servers—
all students—tried to take orders and serve the food as quickly
as possible; they paused only briefly for a chat with residents
and then usually only to make sure the order was taken cor-
rectly.

I was told that residents were offered dinner choices the day
before. From their assigned tables, they were given a list of two
appetizers (salad or soup), three entrées (usually chicken, fish,
or meat), four vegetables, and two desserts (often cake or
kosher ice cream made of soy). They could check off one appe-
tizer, one entrée, two vegetables, and one dessert. But Anne
mentioned that it was quite common for residents to change
their minds, and servers were prepared to oblige, as long as a re-
vised choice was available.

There were five servers for about sixty persons, and they were
polite and friendly—even chummy. But they certainly lacked
serving skills. It wasn't that plates were thrown down on the
table, but they did seem to arrive with a thud as the servers raced
through their duties and, at times, shouted requests to the two
people who set out the individual portions from the warmers.

They also hurried about in response to residents' demands for
prompt service. One resident shouted, "Water! Water!" several
times during the meal; finally another resident handed her own
glass to a server who gave it to the thirsty resident.[3]

My mother and I checked off chicken for an entrée; Aaron
chose pot roast. I noticed that beverage selections included
mostly sodas. I noticed, too, that only generic sodas were available. This turned out to be one of many cost-saving measures
the Glengrove food director had instituted.

Alcoholic drinks were not available, even for purchase.
Aaron and I both like having wine with dinner—and that day
especially I would have enjoyed a glass! I had assumed that
some residents might have liked a glass of wine or beer with
their dinners.

The server, Linda, took our orders and returned with the

meals in a few minutes. "Here you are, sweetie," she said to my mother, who winced at the nickname but thanked her.

The portions were large, and they looked tasty. But they certainly weren't to Aaron's or my liking. They lacked seasoning. I looked for salt on the table, but there wasn't any. In fact, there were no condiments of any kind. "We don't have that sort of thing," said Linda. I later learned that this was a way for Glengrove to better control residents' sodium intake.

As we ate, Alice and my mother engaged in animated conversation, with Alice doing most of the talking. She wanted to know how many pills my mother took each day. The answer: two pills, plus eye drops for glaucoma. "That's nothing," said Alice. "I take eight pills. I have a heart and breathing condition. In the past year, I've been hospitalized three times." The reality I sensed, if Alice was typical of residents, was that most people living at Glengrove had some disabilities or, putting it differently, needed assistance in daily living. Otherwise, they would have been living independently. Indeed, the data seem to indicate that this perception holds for most ALFs.[4]

As we ate, Ira came to the table and introduced his wife, Rachel. They were one of the few couples at Glengrove—and Ira was one of the few men in the dining room. I saw only seven men, five of whom sat at their own tables. The men didn't appear to do much socializing with the women. The prospects of a romance for my mother seemed rather dim. I learned later that Glengrove seemed to have an unwritten policy that discouraged friendships leading to romance, and especially any sexual relations—except for the few married couples.[5]

At one point my mother whispered in my ear, "Look over there." At an adjacent table four diners had brought large doggie bags to the dining room. They asked the servers to wrap up the unused portions of their meals. The servers obliged. The residents seemed to have no hesitancy in making this request. Our server and Alice told us that the bags were a standard procedure at every meal. They said that most of the residents also asked that fresh fruit be included and, again, the servers obliged. My friend Barry, a longtime member of Glengrove's board of directors, suggested that doggie bags were a way for residents to exert greater control over their lives. Others have suggested that because many residents were survivors of World War II, food was both the substance and the symbol of survival.[6]

While we were eating dessert, we heard Cindy, the activities director, on the public address system. Her voice was bubbly, but the tone was that of a kindergarten teacher. She announced that there would be bingo in the social center after dinner. My mother, somewhat to the disappointment of Alice, said that she wanted to go. Alice and Rose, a resident who had once been my mother's neighbor, both said they would join us. "Bingo," Rose said, "is a daily activity at Glengrove."

Before we left the dining room I had a brief chat with Anne. The matter of alcoholic beverages interested me. As I said, I find that a glass of wine makes a meal more pleasant, and I understood that meals were enormously important for most residents. So I asked Anne if there was really a policy restricting alcoholic drinks. "No," she answered, "there's no written policy, but there sure is an informal policy." No drinks of any kind were to be served in the dining room with this exception: On Friday evenings, the start of the Jewish sabbath—Shabbat—all residents were given an ounce of sweet kosher wine as part of the brief ceremony welcoming the sabbath. They were limited to that single one-ounce glass of wine each week.

But did residents have the right to have alcoholic beverages in their apartments? "Of course they do," Anne answered. "However, if we find any resident impaired by alcohol, you can be sure that the matter will come to the attention of Glengrove's resident manager." She explained that a conference between the manager, the resident, and the resident's guarantor might be required. The resident would have to show that he or she would act in a manner appropriate to Glengrove.

Anne's account made the manager at Glengrove seem a bit

like a school principal ordering a student to show cause why discipline should not be meted out. In any event, I wondered why an informal policy that actually seemed quite formal had not been set down in writing so that the residents would be aware of it. Further, wasn't this a subject that a residents' association should consider—and, at the very least, be able to make recommendations to management? I promised myself that I would bend the rules at the party I hoped to give for my mother at Glengrove a few months later when she turned ninety.

Some informal Glengrove policies reflect the formal policies of a government acting in loco parentis. The Canadian Broadcasting Corporation covered a story about the Manitoba Housing Authority's takeover of the management and support of a senior residence in Winnipeg. Authority officials learned that at a Christmas dinner a two-ounce glass of wine was served to each resident who requested it. In fact, for more than twenty years the residents' association had provided a glass of wine at Thanksgiving and Christmas dinners. The residents themselves had collected the money to pay for the wine. Nonetheless, the housing authority announced that the government would end its support for the residents' association and even force its dissolution if the facility continued this service.

It was not clear whether the authority objected in principle to alcohol being served or believed that some of its monies were being used to pay for wine. In any event, soon after news of the authority's actions was broadcast, perhaps in response to public reaction, it rescinded the threatening letter. Wine could be served so long as authority funds were not used.[7]

After finishing our first dinner at Glengrove, we took the elevator to the main floor and walked down the long corridor toward the social center. Along the way I noticed a floor-to-ceiling aviary containing a wide variety of brightly colored little birds. Although glass separated them from watchers, we could hear them chirping, even singing. My mother was enormously taken by them. She walked to the aviary, tapped on the glass and began to chirp herself. Several of the birds seemed to respond. It was a lovely few minutes. I was certain my mother would visit the birds regularly. I later read that the Eden Alternative suggested that ALFs include an aviary or some other way to introduce birds into the assisted living environment.

But our destination now was bingo at the social center. About twenty people from the nursing home, seated for the most part in wheelchairs, already were present with their attending health care aides. An equal number of residents had arrived from the assisted living facility. For the most part the ALF residents seemed to keep apart from those in the nursing home.

The volunteers passed out bingo cards. Ruby, the volunteer who called the numbers, reminded the players: "Remember, this is just like all of our bingo games. Everyone, at some point, will win. Each winner will get twenty-five cents." The play began and volunteers circulated to make sure numbers were blocked off. They were patient and helpful. The players got involved in the games, and they seemed especially pleased to win. For Alice, however, the game was a painful bore, though she stayed until my mother had won her twenty-five cents.

For those who didn't win, the volunteers, their aprons filled with change, walked around about an hour later and dispensed a quarter to each player. Aaron and I didn't qualify, because we were guests. This much can be said of bingo: It is a way of passing time.[8]

We walked back to the residence, my mother chirping goodnight as we passed the birds. I was tired, and I think that even my usually energetic son was weary. My mother, however, seemed revitalized. Rose, who lived on the ground floor, left us at her apartment. Alice asked my mother if she would like to visit her for a little while. The answer was a quick "Yes!"

Alice and my mother walked with Aaron and me to the entrance. It was only about 7:30, but the building was utterly quiet. There were neither residents nor aides on the floor. My mother noticed that the front office was dark. "Where is the security for this place?" she asked. Alice, in turn, asked my mother what she meant. After all, Alice said, no one could get in. The automatic doors at the entrance were locked, and one could only get access by an outside buzzer connected with the nursing home. An audio intercom required people seeking entrance to identify themselves. If the employee was satisfied, an entrance buzzer was sounded and the door opened. It was clear that my mother was not satisfied with this level of security. Aaron and I said good-night. Alice and my mother headed toward the elevator, continuing their conversation. On the whole, I thought it had been a good first day.

I was relieved that my mother seemed to be making new friends and appeared to be settling into her new home, yet I wondered at the lack of any sort of orientation. It was a sentiment my mother later echoed when she said, "It would be nice if there could be a welcoming committee to greet new residents." She raised that point with Susan, the residence manager, who agreed but said she just didn't have the time. My mother then raised the point with the residents' association at its regular monthly meeting. The residents listened, as did Cindy, the activities director, and the CEO of Glengrove, who usually came to the association meetings. It wasn't that the idea was rejected. It simply wasn't acted upon.

When I thought about the lack of any sort of orientation at the facility, I was reminded of Aaron who, as a child, was scheduled to have a tonsillectomy at Toronto's Hospital for Sick Children, a world-class facility. Though acting bravely, he clearly was worried about the procedure. Then came a letter from the hospital addressed to Aaron. He was invited with his parents to visit the hospital in advance of his surgery—to see what was involved, and to meet those who would care for him.

We went to the hospital at the assigned time. A registered nurse greeted us and introduced herself. She told us she would be Aaron's nurse both before and after the surgery. Next we went to a lecture room where there were about twenty other children scheduled for the same procedure. A surgeon and anesthesiologist who would be performing the procedure spoke briefly, intelligently, and respectfully to the children, and answered the few questions they posed. Finally, the nurse took us to the recovery room where she explained to Aaron how he would probably feel after the surgery, and promised him ice cream. This, I thought, was a helpful orientation. So did Aaron.

If we can do this for small children, why can't ALFs do it for elderly residents? That is why my mother suggested creating a greeting committee. She wanted to help new residents feel more comfortable in what they thought was to be a home for the rest of their lives.

Life at Glengrove was defined in no small measure by the institution and those who served it. The way the institution defined itself placed constraints on residents, restrictions that neither my mother nor I investigated. The residents might have chosen—as did my mother and I—to turn a blind eye on the "sick building," the units for skilled nursing care, and the nursing home. But these facilities were part of Glengrove, just as they are in many assisted living facilities.[9]

Wouldn't it have been better if the residents were taken to visit the skilled nursing units and the nursing home so that they could understand Glengrove's promise of aging in place? Surely their existence raised a question—and a fear—in many ALF residents: if they became impaired after a fall, for example, would they really be able to age in place? Could they remain in their apartments, and if so, under what conditions? Could they make plans that would allow them to stay? Or would they be placed without their consent in a skilled care unit, later to be transferred to a room in the nursing home?

In fact the skilled nursing unit and the nursing home, while physically a part of Glengrove, could be accessed only by elevator, which tended to be restrictive to those who were impaired. However, volunteers, family members or other visitors often brought many of those cared for in these units to the deli.

Parts of the residents' handbook confused me. For example, it stated that residents could stay in their apartments so long as they could function independently. But residents and their families could see that many residents were already in wheelchairs or used walkers, and others suffered from a moderate level of dementia. Still others hired aides (called "companions") who helped them with daily needs ranging from dressing to toileting.

Had there been open discussion between management and residents during a real orientation, residents might have posed this important question: Will we be able to stay in our apartments, as we lose capacity, so long as we are not a danger to ourselves or others? Management's answer would have helped me and other family members as well as our parents determine how to maximize what independence was left to them. At the very least it would have defined the limitations of aging in place.

An orientation might also have given my mother and I the opportunity to meet the staff. It was the staff—that is, the health care aides—who actualized institutional policy. The critical senior staff members were Susan, manager of the Glengrove ALF residences; Bee, the licensed practical nurse; Cindy, the activities director; and Anne, the dining room manager.

On move-in day we saw people pushing linen carts in the hallways. Who were they? No one in management told us. It was Alice who said they were health care aides. These were the people who did the beds, vacuumed the rugs, dusted, loaded the dishwasher, and sometimes helped residents dress or move about. Several aides smiled at us. But sometime later Alice whispered, "Almost all of them will be gone in a few months. They don't stay very long." That may be why there were no introductions.

As I'll describe more fully in the next chapter, staff retention was a problem for Glengrove, just as it has been for other ALFs and nursing homes. Staff turnover in any one year nationally runs from 50 percent to almost 100 percent. And this turnover relates not just to the least-skilled and the lowest-paid employees, the health care aides, but to senior staff and management.[10]

A few months into my mother's stay at Glengrove, Cindy, employed for less than two years there, was already looking for another job, one closer to her home. The Glengrove chief executive officer, employed for only six months, was about to be discharged. Susan, a stalwart senior employee who had been with the Orthodox home for more than twenty years, was in the process of being transferred to rent to potential residents forty new, smaller units from what had been Glengrove's Alzheimer wing. Known as "the Gardens," these were moderately priced one-room units, which my mother referred to as the "peanut apartments." (The Alzheimer patients had been moved to enclosed quarters on the second floor of the nursing home.)

For residents of Glengrove and other ALFs, a close relationship with the staff has a special importance. That closeness gives residents a sense of stability within a changing community. Initially neither my mother nor I gave this obvious fact any thought. We never asked about turnover or staff ratios and retention. My mother was in good health, she was making new friends at Glengrove, and she had a firm base of outside support. She didn't think much about her dependence on paid professionals or aides. But later in her stay at Glengrove, the high turnover of the staff would affect us both.

3 The Early Years at Glengrove

THE SETTING

When my mother moved in, Glengrove seemed to be a pleasant, welcoming environment. My mother was eighty-nine at the time, but the average age for admission to Glengrove, like that of most ALFs, was eighty-two. Most of the residents had some physical disabilities, but all new residents had passed tests (taken without their knowledge) to show that they could function relatively independently—even if that meant using a walker or having the partial assistance of a wheelchair. They were, on the whole, mobile and mentally alert. Glengrove, like other ALFs, accepted physical handicaps but could less easily cope with residents who were mentally disoriented or, as my mother said, had "lost it."

Glengrove did not sell itself as caring for the "frailest of the frail," but it did take residents in the middle or later stages of Alzheimer's disease or dementia. These residents lived in a separate unit referred to as the "rementia" unit, adjacent to the nursing home and staffed on a 24/7 basis by nurses, including registered nurses, as required by state law. "Rementia" is a term used by many ALFs as a positive label for dealing with dementia and relates to learning and experiencing cognitive clarity despite degenerative cognitive impairment. (It would be difficult for residents and family—even staff—to have a unit called the "dementia unit.") Generally, unless in the company of staff or family, rementia residents did not socialize with ALF residents.

Had we visited Glengrove four years after its doors had opened, the picture would have been very different. Residents would have been moving out of apartments to the nursing home; they would have had increased levels of disabilities; and more would have been dying.

When my mother first arrived at Glengrove, the facility seemed to deliver what its advertising and marketing promised—a homelike environment where the staff focus was on meeting the challenges of daily life rather than decline.[1] And at the start of her new journey, and for the first three years of her residency, she was a relatively healthy elderly person living with other relatively healthy elderly people. But later the lines became less clear to her as her own abilities began to lessen.

A MODEL RESIDENT

Through visits and phone calls to the resident manager, the head of volunteers, and friends and relatives who visited with my mother on a regular basis, I kept tabs on how she was doing. I wanted to get a fix on the quality of her life and to spot any difficulties early on and deal with them, if she was not able to do so herself. If, for example, she had a disagreement with a resident—and this did happen—that of course was for her to resolve. I did not want to intrude.

In her own way, my mother fashioned a world where there was life, hope, and a measure of stability. To a considerable extent, it was a world that was largely, though not totally, open to me and her friends and family. But there were some residents who quite clearly had isolated themselves. One could see it in their expressionless faces and slumped bodies. My mother was not one of them.

It seemed to me that my mother's first three years at Glengrove were good for her and for Glengrove as well. Residents like my mother make it possible for such ALFs to remain largely occupied without filling empty apartments with the frail.

My mother was undemanding, even helpful, to staff and

other residents. During the first part of her residency, she required little staff attention. Except for some positive suggestions to the activities director—such as recommending a Chinese restaurant where the food was good and the price was low as a place for an ALF luncheon outing—and pleasant chats with the then manager of the apartments, her only deep and ongoing contacts were with the volunteers and with Susan, who was both the apartment manager and a social worker, and Cindy, the activities director.

When she first took up residence, my mother quickly developed a rapport with Susan and Cindy. They became her friends. She continued to see Sol Shapiro, who had become her doctor after Walter Gold's death. Unlike most of the residents' physicians, he did not require patients to come to his office for appointments; he visited them.

Sol was a member of Glengrove's board of directors, and he often visited my mother in her new home. Many of his visits were not to see her as a patient but to try to get her impressions about how the new facility was doing. My mother felt that she was involved, that she had input. She wanted to be of assistance. The staff was there to help her and others, but she was there to help the staff as well. At one point she was even allowed into the kitchen to show the chef how to make "proper brisket."

My mother's cooking and baking were helpful social tools. Quite selectively, she gave small samples of her prized strudel to potential friends. From time to time, she would make latkes. As they were frying, the aroma of potatoes, garlic, and onions would reach the hall. She said there often were knocks on her door from residents who wondered what she was cooking. Often, they were invited in to share some of what they had smelled.

In many ways, my mother seemed freer and happier than she had been in years. Her days in the past had been full, but she recognized that she was now at a new stage of life—and this included living each day fully.

Glengrove's bus regularly took residents, at no additional charge, to shopping areas, including trips to supermarkets. The drivers were full-time employees who generally had warm feelings for the residents that went beyond merely transporting them. Often, when my mother was not feeling well and stayed in her apartment, a driver would buy her small packages of licorice, her favorite candy, as presents. And the drivers, as well as the activities director, were patient with the residents, who frequently were not at the loading area at departure time. Seldom did any scheduled trip leave on time. Where possible, outings were scheduled around the needs of the residents.

On her shopping trips, my mother often bought new clothes —primarily to wear at the Sunday concerts held for both the ALF and the nursing home. Small groups or bands played and sang. The residents of the apartments seemed to see my mother as part of the entertainment, and for that matter so did many of the patients of the nursing home brought by volunteers. Soon after the music began, my mother danced—alone—and as she danced, she smiled, said hello, and shook the hands of residents who reached out to her.

In all my years I had never seen my mother dance. To my surprise, she told me that, as a young woman, she had taught dancing before she was married. A niece married a year after my mother entered Glengrove. We went to the wedding. There, I danced with my mother—and so did a number of young men. On reflection, I think what my mother had done was to take an unrehearsed part in the entertainment at Glengrove. At most ALF activities residents were passive observers waiting to be entertained, but she had taken control. It was a wonderful sight.

My mother got a thrill seeing how other residents responded to her. She seemed to catch their imagination. I saw women residents with walkers dance to the music, wave, and shake hands. Still, I didn't see the staff or management encourage the residents to be creative beyond taking part in what they, the staff, had put in place, such as a fashion show where resident volunteers—including my mother—modeled clothes. In fact, sometimes the entertainment chosen was mildly unsettling to residents, who were adults, not children.

One Sunday concert featured Jack's Talent School, a group of children aged eight to twelve who demonstrated their acquired talent—sometimes to their own obvious irritation but to the pride of their parents. In a particularly excruciating performance, an eleven-year-old boy played "jazz" on a piano. He looked utterly bored and made the simple piece, which should have been short, painfully long.

Sitting next to me, in a wheelchair, was Stan Saath, once an accomplished jazz pianist. I had enjoyed listening to him tickle out a few tunes on the grand piano in the lobby when there had been only a few listeners and he felt relatively comfortable. Stan grimaced as he listened to the unwilling child play. I fantasized that Glengrove could have initiated some sort of program in which residents like Stan could mentor a willing child, even playing with him. But by then I had learned that nothing like that was likely to happen.

My mother also went to a number of stage shows outside the facility as part of Glengrove's outing plan. When we had initially heard that residents could be taken to these events, my mother balked at the expense. When I bought her a subscription, she changed her mind. She enjoyed herself and talked about the plays.

My mother was seldom in her apartment. Her new answering machine became a contact point for friends and relatives, including friends at Glengrove. She quickly learned to push the right buttons for what to her was a novel technology.

Shortly after her arrival, my mother seemed to become a poster person. Her picture was taken many times and used in advertisements for Glengrove in the local Jewish newspaper. My cousin Herb, then living in Florida, subscribed to the newspaper. He became a clipping service of my mother's doings. She was aware of the articles, but modesty stopped her from mentioning them to me—so I mentioned them to her and suggested that, with her popularity, she consider running for city council in the small community where Glengrove was located. I was serious about the suggestion, but my mother replied that she was busy enough!

Glengrove's managers also viewed her apartment as a model. When the staff wanted to show potential tenants or visiting state inspectors a model furnished apartment—and a model tenant—they often selected my mother and her apartment. This gave her pleasure.

My mother and Alice, her best friend and next-door neighbor, became inseparable. More than once my mother told me, "Alice is more than a friend. She's a sister." They argued from time to time, and even stopped talking with each other for a day or two. But they were bonded and got together again. They wanted, perhaps even needed, each other's company.

Yet they did seem an unusual pair. Alice, in her eighties, was large, brassy, and quick to judgment. My mother was petite, quiet, and, more often than not, restrained. "It's better not to say anything about people around here," my mother said. "They do tend to gossip." Alice had chronic ailments ranging from a heart condition to respiratory problems. She took several medications and used a walker. Only a few relatives, her distant cousins, visited her. She seldom saw her son, who lived in San Diego, though she often spoke of him.

Alice was alert and intelligent. She scoffed at those residents who, in her view, only ate and slept. After dinner she, my mother, and residents invited to join them played Scrabble in the library. Then, after about an hour, my mother and Alice adjourned to Alice's apartment, where they watched her large television set and talked. Alice, who handled her own finances through a trust, helped my mother balance her checkbook and write checks. This was helpful because my mother's eyesight was deteriorating rapidly.

Alice had come to Glengrove from another ALF, and she thought that her new home was better by far. During her first three years as a resident, she kept her large car, with scarcely any mileage, in a little-used section of Glengrove's parking lot reserved for residents. Alice said that she kept the car because of the feeling of freedom that it gave her. From time to time she drove around the parking area. (My mother chose not to be a passenger.) In her third year at Glengrove, she sold the car to the son of her cousin. It was the same year that she had a representative of a funeral home visit her and then made arrangements for her funeral. Alice asked my mother if she wanted to do the same for herself. My mother said no.

Alice's age and poor health put her relationship with my mother on a fragile, but enduring, foundation. For Alice, however, the chief concern was not her own health but my mother's. On more than one occasion, Alice telephoned me, concerned about my mother's condition, which ranged from not eating to having a cold. About herself Alice said nothing, at least not to me. My mother, on the other hand, frequently said of Alice: "She's one sick girl." Several times, according to my mother, staff at Glengrove called 911 for an ambulance to take Alice to a nearby hospital for emergency treatment.

My mother made other friends, though none as close as Alice. They included Rachel, who was eighty-seven and had moved to Glengrove at about the same time. Rachel joined my mother and Alice in their after-dinner Scrabble games. She had no close relatives, though on occasion a cousin came to visit. Unlike Alice, Rachel often seemed depressed. She discussed her problems with my mother, who became her confidante. Many of those problems were financial. At one level, Rachel's situation seemed very like my mother's. She had owned, mortgage-free, a modest home which she sold for about sixty thousand dollars. Like my mother, she had worked most of her adult life, qualifying her for a modest monthly pension of $175 and Social Security benefits. But unlike my mother, she had no relatives to supplement what turned out, by Glengrove's standards, to be meager assets.

Nonetheless, Rachel applied for an apartment, and she was welcomed because the chair of the facility's board of directors was striving for full occupancy to increase cash flow. Rachel disclosed her financial situation, but no one seemed to question it. Glengrove didn't ask a social worker to explore the possible availability of welfare programs that might provide rent subsidies. Perhaps the management calculated that, statistically, she wouldn't be around very long. Rachel was given a one-bedroom apartment. She paid her rent on time, and until her money ran out, things seemed to go well for her and for the friendship that she formed with Alice and my mother.

My mother did not anticipate any of the serious financial problems that Rachel would experience. Nor did she see in Alice's deteriorating health a warning about her own future. Instead, for at least the first three years she seemed excited with her new home at Glengrove.

A BIRTHDAY PARTY

My mother's ninetieth birthday came two months after she entered Glengrove. I asked her if she would like a party. She said no, arguing that all her friends—except for Alice and Rachel—and most of her relatives of her age were dead. I answered that a party probably could be held at Glengrove in the cultural center where the Sunday concerts took place. Tables could be set up for a nice, simple brunch. I knew a piano player who could play while people dined and sing songs my mother enjoyed. He had appeared at several Sunday concerts at Glengrove. I asked my mother to think about it and simply write down the names of people she might want to invite. We could give it a few weeks.

My mother gave it some thought. At the end of one of our telephone chats, she said that perhaps she would like to have a party. She had drawn up a "little guest list." Apparently, all her friends and most of her relatives had not died. There were sixty names, and by the time of the party the list had increased to about eighty. When she asked if I minded that she had gone over sixty, I told her I didn't mind at all.

Among those invited was Aunt Lil, two years younger than my mother. Aunt Lil lived in Palm Springs, California. A high-energy person as outspoken as Alice, she still drove her car, wore high heels, and was a sharp player of gin rummy and bridge. Aunt Lil agreed to visit my mother in what became the start of a tradition of two visits a year. I purchased a book of senior air tickets; Cousin Herb made the reservations. Cousins who lived in the area picked up Aunt Lil at the airport, and she stayed at Glengrove with my mother. Her encounters with Alice were lively, to say the least, with my mother in the background, enjoying their banter, often chuckling.

Glengrove's chef, as he preferred to be called, was able to accommodate us for the birthday brunch. Once again my mother managed to penetrate the sanctum of the kitchen, where she was invited to show him how to make a few dishes that she thought the guests would enjoy.

I thought this would be a good time to break the wine barrier. So I ordered two cases of wine that I knew was kosher because it came from a kosher store and was so labeled. But I had not before encountered the Orthodox rabbi who, as a primary duty, inspected food and drink for kosher observance. "There's kosher and kosher," he said. For reasons I could not comprehend, the wine I ordered was not sufficiently kosher. I asked the rabbi to order the wine, and he agreed. As it turned out, with the Orthodox rabbi looking on, no more than a few bottles of wine were served to the eighty guests, and the residents consumed only a handful of glasses. But at least I had the satisfaction of serving wine to residents at Glengrove.

Ira, the president of the newly formed residents' association, asked if he and others could sing a Hebrew song—loosely translated as "How Good It Is for Friends to Dwell Together"—that they, along with my mother, had learned for the recent dedication of the new facilities at Glengrove. Later, when the cake was carried in, my mother announced that she had a few words to say. With a big smile, she said she had a wish: she asked if there could be a party the next year. I promised her that there would be—and there was.

The party, I thought, was splendid. My mother had a glow about her. The next day, however, Susan called me aside. "The party was great," she said, "but if you plan to do this next year, something will have to change. A lot people among the residents were not invited, and they feel hurt. In the future, if there's to be a party at Glengrove, why not have a big birthday cake and ice cream for everyone in the lobby?"

I listened to Susan with some concern. My understanding had been that my mother was going to live independently. She was perfectly capable of making decisions for herself. I was determined that she should decide between a birthday cake in the lobby and a party off-site. If the party were held away from Glengrove—as it was for two birthdays—then Glengrove's bus could transport guests. If the party were held at Glengrove—as was the case for two other birthdays—then the lobby could be decorated with balloons and there could be a small band playing my mother's favorite tunes. Birthday decisions were no easy matter.

INTIMACY AT GLENGROVE

My post–birthday party conversation with Susan raised some issues. It seemed there were unwritten rules and assumptions that no one had conveyed to residents and their families. One was about social events; another was about intimacy between residents. My mother, who generally didn't gossip, told me of a romance between two residents. Sex, it seemed, was off limits. The couple subsequently moved to an apartment elsewhere and apparently never returned to visit Glengrove.

Intimacy is an aspect of life that ALFs treat differently. At

Glengrove, residents understood that sex was unacceptable, and there were no engagements or marriages during my mother's years there. Glengrove's unwritten rules, however, vary sharply from those of a scattering of other ALFs, such as the Hebrew Home for the Aged, a facility in the Bronx with about 1,100 residents and a staff of 2,000. There, sex among the aging is not considered taboo, and the ALF staff is instructed accordingly. One day, when a housekeeping aide at the Home softly knocked on an apartment door and there was no answer, she opened it and found a couple, each of whom had Alzheimer's, having sex. She quietly said, "Excuse me," shut the door, and made a mental note to come back later to clean the apartment.

"We understand that sex is the outgrowth of intimacy, affection, and caring," said Daniel Reingold, executive vice president of the Home. "Our goal is to encourage those emotions while also being aware of the rights and safety of others."[2]

It is somewhat unclear just what "rights and safety of others" means. Reingold suggested that if family members find out and object to a parent having sex, the home likely would put a damper on such activity. With the cooperation of doctors, sexual activity could be inhibited by prescribing drugs that dampen the sexual urge. This, of course, raises other issues. Why do family members have the right to curtail the sex lives of people who have obviously been having sexual relations throughout their adult lives?

Some ALFs insist that they must protect residents who have medical problems that, in their view, could be exacerbated by sexual activity. At an ALF located in Bethesda, Maryland, when the child of a resident became aware that her father was having sex and complained that he might have "a stroke or something," an administrator responded that then he would "go out with a smile." The reality, for this administrator at least, is that sex exists and age is no barrier.

Some ALFs, even those dealing with residents with moderate dementia, issue codes of conduct to their staffs which "respect the intimacy of residents." But so far the number of such ALFs is small.

Of course, there are times when both the state and the facility's management may intrude into residents' sex lives. For example, a state can view sex with someone suffering from severe dementia as sexual assault because, as one police officer put it, how can such persons give their consent? Further, the ALF may well lose its right to continue to operate because it has failed to "protect" the residents, as required by state law.

Intimacy is not an experience that all elderly residents will embrace. Some will not do so because of the era in which they were raised. Others may not because, as one female resident of a Florida senior community explained it, there are few incentives for female residents to make the first move on the available men in the community. "Look, the men are old and decrepit," she said. "That is what you are dealing with here. And let's face it: men my age, they don't want me. The men are either looking for a nurse or a purse."[3]

Some residents may be wary of getting too close to other people. Friendships can be fleeting. It's no easy matter to say good-bye to special friends made at the ALF—a fact my mother later experienced when Alice died.

OTHER ACTIVITIES AND MONEY

For those who chose to steer clear of romantic entanglements, there were activities besides bingo. Some were one-time events, such as when (at the suggestion of Glengrove's CEO) my mother, Alice, and other residents raised funds for a park memorial to Israeli soldiers. Once they obtained the funds, a memorial service was held in which a choir, including my mother and Alice, participated.

Each week at Glengrove, the activities director, who had a modest budget but seldom consulted residents about their wishes (except regarding lunches at nearby restaurants), scheduled institutional activities. These were announced in large-type handouts that were tacked up on bulletin boards and also placed in small baskets mounted beside each resident's door.

Residents usually signed up for outings, such as theater. The cost of the outings was borne by the residents, who had to pay in advance. A ticket price of more than a few dollars was a real disincentive for residents, most of whom seemed to have a deep fear of not having enough money. The activities that produced the largest turnout were inexpensive lunches that cost about five dollars or a ride on Glengrove's bus on summer days to look at the scenery and stop for ice cream.

Neither the actual budget allocation nor proposed budgets were vetted with the residents, or for that matter with the activities director herself. Glengrove's CEO simply told her the amount of her budget.

Rental movies were shown at Glengrove twice weekly, though my mother rejected this as an activity after seeing the first. Her reason: too much violence and sex. It was a PG-rated film.

The event most frequently scheduled at Glengrove, and probably most ALFs, was bingo, held several times a week. It brought residents together socially for chatter and activity—and that was no small benefit. The game seemed to encourage a certain social hierarchy. Seating was not random: it was expected that friends would sit together and that newcomers would find their own way.[4]

Every few months Glengrove's bus took apartment residents to a riverboat casino. These outings, which began at noon, seemed to heighten the adrenaline and pleasure levels of the residents. The casino had a buffet, which my mother said was generous, tasty, and cost only five dollars. Like most of the residents, my mother went to the twenty-five-cent slots. She didn't go to just any available machine. Rather, she scouted them to get an idea of which seemed to pay more frequently. She decided that the machines near the entrance were the ones to play. "Probably," she said, "they put them there so that people coming in will think all the machines pay off a lot."

On any outing she never took more than ten dollars in quarters. If she lost the full amount, that was the end of gambling for the day. It seemed, however, that my mother was a winner most of the time, and she never lost her ten-dollar stake. The same was not true for all residents, she said. "Many of them lost as much as seventy-five dollars. And that was money they couldn't afford." Apparently, some families complained to the administration, and the casino outings became less frequent, although Glengrove itself sponsored a benefit casino night for contributors to the institution.

There were some events involving little cost that gave my mother and other residents pleasure and, it seemed, a start for new relationships. In the first year of her residence, holiday exchange programs were developed with a nearby Christian ALF, only a ten-minute walk from Glengrove. Christian residents came to Glengrove, where residents together with the Reform rabbi explained and enacted services for Jewish holidays such as Passover. The same was done for Christian holidays. Perhaps just as meaningful was the opportunity for the residents of the two facilities to talk with one another.

The activities directors of the two ALFs launched the programs. When Glengrove's activities director resigned within her first year, the exchange program was not continued. Apparently, the residents of Glengrove, who seemed to quite enjoy the program, either did not feel they had the power to carry the exchange forward or believed that they lacked the means to do so. After all, some institutional involvement was required. Because many residents were not fully ambulatory, a bus was needed to make the short trip between the institutions. Further, there had to be some coordination with the kitchen of each facility since the holidays frequently involved food.

A VOICE FOR THE RESIDENTS

Residents of Glengrove, like those of other ALFs, did have some means for making their views known. Individually, they often spoke with the residence manager or the activities director, offering suggestions or making complaints. In the final analysis, however, any resulting action depended on the goodwill of the manager or activities director. When it came to issues such as rent increases or staffing difficulties, management rarely solicited the input of residents.

There were, at least on the surface, other more formal ways for residents to express themselves. Glengrove formed an association to provide residents with a voice. However, the residents' association seldom confronted management or put forward issues to negotiate. Whether the residents feared reprisals or were inexperienced in dealing with institutional hierarchy, I do not know. But I did sense that the residents seemed to believe that the facility belonged not to them but to those who ran it. Yet, who in fact does run a not-for-profit assisted living facility? Why, even if control lies outside the residents, can they not have meaningful input into decision making that affects their lives?[5]

When my mother first came to Glengrove, the dining room staff consisted of young people, most of whom were students. They might have lacked the polish of professional servers, but they quickly developed a warmth for the residents, who responded in kind. My mother frequently asked some to run errands for her at the end of their shifts, and they willingly obliged.

One day, about a year later, the entire dining room serving staff was dismissed without notice. That same day, they were replaced by another group, somewhat fewer in number but equally pleasant. What I found strange was that the residents said nothing about the change. They asked no questions. Management volunteered no information and solicited no views from residents. And the residents made no inquiries as to where their favorite servers had gone, except perhaps among themselves.

The residents' association had elected officers. It held monthly meetings, which most residents attended. The activities director took notes. The association had no income; it charged no dues and received no funds from Glengrove or any other source.

A past president of the residents' association said that Glengrove's CEO had told her that each meeting was to last at least an hour. Often, she said, that was difficult to achieve. Seldom was there either old or new business. Though the residents came to the meetings with concerns, she said, they seldom voiced them.

So what took place at the meetings? The past president said that department heads spent much of the required hour delivering operational reports. It was a kind of verbal billboard that expanded on what the activities director had earlier posted. No operational report was made concerning the dismissal of the dining room staff.

The single subject that did attract considerable resident comment was food. About this topic there was no resident shyness or acceptance of management prerogative. Dining was a central feature of a resident's day. It was a time for them to socialize and, they hoped, enjoy some good cooking. Lunch and dinner were served at specific times and seldom was anyone late. Many lined up in front of the dining room up to a half hour before meals were served. Walkers and wheelchairs abounded. The dining room manager had a central role in orchestrating each meal.

High-end ALFs advertised what they called their quality dining facilities. Glengrove was no exception. But from my experience on my mother's moving day and the many meals that followed, I certainly didn't think that the food served deserved a high rating. But perhaps what I prefer in food, such as moist fish and medium-rare meat, would not have appealed to the residents or the chef-nutritionist concerned about resident health. For the most part, the chefs at Glengrove did not seem to last long—only a matter of months.

Parties held in the cultural center—marking, for example, religious holidays—were attended by residents, nursing home patients, and outside guests. On these occasions the quality and variety of food ranged between good and excellent. But the daily fare was usually bland and served lukewarm or cold.

My mother's response to food she didn't like was simple: she left the dining room, went to her apartment and prepared something she did like, such as chicken livers laced with onion or sweet-and-sour cabbage. This was not the practice of most residents, though I once fantasized just such a mass response to a particularly bad meal.

The residents' association was not permitted to discuss food, I was told. That role was assigned to an all-inclusive Glengrove food committee. Most residents attended its monthly meetings. I could not understand the difference between the association and this committee. The food services manager was present and he usually brought a large notebook. The residents spoke, and he appeared to be recording carefully what they were saying. Comments and complaints were forthcoming from the residents.

At dinner one night in the dining room, Mrs. Solomon, a past president of the residents' association, spoke to me with some pride about what the food committee had achieved after months of discussion with management. She asked me if I noticed anything different on the tables from my previous visit. I did. On each table were containers of catsup and mustard. The residents, she said, really had to argue long and hard for these condiments.

Anne supervised the dining room staff while keeping her eyes on the residents, ready to help when needed. At a table near where I sat on a visit with my mother, I noticed a woman who would not lift her arms up toward her food. She had some sores on her arms. Anne approached the resident quietly and gently placed some bandages on the affected areas. Then the woman ate. A man, mildly palsied, spilled his drink. Anne quickly covered the wet spot with a napkin so that he could continue eating.

Anne and Susan always seemed sensitive to the residents and what they saw as the residents' best interests, even in the face of occasional anger and shouting. The food committee and the residents' association, in their view, were shallow. They had little time for what they saw as form without substance. They did have time, or made time, for the concerns of any individual resident.

THE VOLUNTEERS

Volunteers, mostly women in their sixties, staffed the deli, a large, brightly lit area with many small tables and chairs. It had the same food as most urban delis (all kosher) though without necessarily the same flavor or mountainous portions. Yet, whatever it might have lacked in taste or serving size, it made up for with personalities.

When my mother first came to Glengrove, Simon, a man in his mid-eighties with a husky, booming voice, dominated the deli. He was a World War II survivor who had escaped the Nazi onslaught in his native Poland by hiding in the woods near peasant villages. To survive, he scavenged onions from neighboring fields. Simon liked to talk, and he seemed to have a special affinity for my mother, who walked to the deli on most days. Usually my mother would only order a half sandwich, at half the price. But at least when I was visiting, Simon managed to place the filling for a whole sandwich into her smaller order.

Jimmy, a thin, rather elegant-looking volunteer in his seventies, usually served my mother, as well as others who could not easily come to the counter and then carry the food to their tables. Within two years, both Simon and Jimmy were gone. Simon told me he was going to have surgery. Although he anticipated a good outcome, he died a few days after the procedure. Jimmy married a disabled woman of means and left the deli to take care of his new wife. Alice suggested that Jimmy may have married for money. My mother said nothing.

Sylvia, an avid golfer probably in her early sixties, was a longtime volunteer who had worked at the old Orthodox home. She seemed to be at the deli several hours each day, four days a week, always wearing her apron. After Simon was gone Sylvia filled in behind the counter, taking orders, making sandwiches, and handling the cash. When she wasn't there, she was visiting the bedridden in the nursing home, talking with people in the deli, or helping with the bingo games.

I learned later that Sylvia and her sister, who also was a volunteer, were quite wealthy. The two had established a foundation to support residents and patients at Glengrove. Diminutive like my mother, Sylvia was gentle with the residents but assertive with staff and Glengrove officials. If there were problems with the bureaucracy, Sylvia often knew the right person to speak to.

The volunteers were a force to contend with. When the merged institution that became Glengrove was in the planning stage, a group of them, at their own expense, inspected a number of other nonprofit ALFs, including the world-class Baycrest facility run by the Jewish community in Toronto. These volunteers tried to have their ideas included in the final planning of Glengrove, and they wanted to have an ongoing role in improving the quality of life of residents and patients. To some extent they succeeded. They raised more than $250,000 for a main-floor Alzheimer's wing that had an outside garden designed so residents could safely wander through it. There was also an interior crafts room. The wing lasted only a matter of months. Because of the need for revenue, these were the units senior management ordered be converted to the single-room suites, the ones my mother referred to as the peanut apartments.

The volunteers continued to raise money and keep in contact with the residents both in the ALF and the nursing home. They formed close personal ties with residents and were aware of their ups and downs. They responded when a resident was worried that friends and family might not be visiting often enough or failed to pick them up for an outing. Sylvia once told me that after Alice died, a group of volunteers saw my mother alone and depressed. They asked her if she would like to go with them to a pops concert downtown. She agreed. After the concert, they took her for a late-evening treat—a hamburger with onions. The evening gave my mother a lift.

MINISTERS (RABBIS AND CHAPLAINS)

The Orthodox and Reform rabbis, both young, worked on a part-time basis. They were paid for a twenty-four-hour week, which meant that Glengrove had put a salary cap on what each rabbi would earn. If the rabbis spent more time with residents, they weren't reimbursed.

I say "rabbi," but during the first two years of my mother's stay at Glengrove, the person who filled that position on the Reform side (which was attended by most of the residents) was a rabbinic student. She was a warm, outgoing person, and the residents respectfully referred to her as Rabbi Sandy. In spite of her salary cap, she was always present on the Friday night Shabbat and the Saturday service, as well as other holidays.

Rabbi Sandy stayed until she was ordained, and then she visited often. She was succeeded by Rabbi Nathan, a jovial, welcoming man who preferred to devote much of the Sabbath service to talking with residents and asking about their week. Although he recited the requisite Jewish prayers and read from the Torah, he used their experiences as a point of departure to tell traditional Jewish stories.

One might have expected competition between the Orthodox and Reform rabbis, but this was not the case. At times they officiated together. They seemed to be on relatively friendly terms, and the Orthodox rabbi, who was steeped in the study of the Torah, even helped Rabbi Sandy with her own studies leading to ordination.

When it came to certain questions, the Orthodox rabbi had the last word. He had the right to declare and enforce Glengrove's dietary regulations, which governed what food residents could eat and how it would be cooked and served.

The chief Orthodox rabbi in the area where Glengrove was

located was the final arbiter in any disputed food matter. In fact, however, he was seldom seen at Glengrove, and so far as I could determine, matters in dispute seldom reached him for decision. He did appear at the Glengrove opening for a walk-through.

Management supported the informality of the Reform rabbis. Rabbi Nathan had a golden retriever, a gentle, friendly dog who was never on a leash and who even attended religious services. The rabbi monitored the dog carefully, but it never barked, never jumped on any resident, and always liked to be petted. As part of the Eden Alternative Movement, Glengrove encouraged this.

Rabbi Nathan also brought his sons, aged three and four when he first began to serve at Glengrove. Unlike the dog, they liked to jump and run through the halls. Without exception, the residents smiled and enjoyed their company. At times Rabbi Nathan, when visiting a grieving or ailing resident, would leave his boys with my mother, who, like other residents, enjoyed being with children. But my mother imposed certain rules, such as not jumping on her furniture. Bribed by some of her strudel, the boys usually complied. Over the years, as the rabbi's sons grew older, they continued to relate easily with the residents.

Unlike residents of ALFs that don't have chaplains, residents at Glengrove—particularly those coping with a serious sickness, an injury, or the death of a loved one—were given spiritual guidance. The rabbis helped to shape a community, and their presence seemed to bring a certain comfort to those attending at prayers, including the Kaddish, the prayer affirming belief and remembering the dead.

In his conversations, Rabbi Nathan often referred to himself as a chaplain. He seemed to be underlining the distinction between someone employed by an institution to serve the needs of its residents and a rabbi chosen by a congregation and serving at their will. He understood that the residents had no input into the selection of their rabbi and could not define his or her role. In fact, Rabbi Nathan told me that it was the CEO of Glengrove who hired him, after interviews not with the residents but with a committee of the board of directors. His responsibility was to his "boss," as he put it, which made his job difficult since no CEO seemed to last long.[6]

The job indeed was difficult. Consider that Glengrove had sixty apartment residents, forty small-unit residents, and more than a hundred nursing home patients. Most residents would become more needy as years passed. The illness and death of family members and new friends at Glengrove would occur with greater frequency. Could one part-time rabbi ever minister to all those in need?

Rabbi Friedman, founding director of Chaplaincy Services at the Philadelphia Geriatric Center, raised the possibility of starting a "para-chaplaincy" program which would likely involve volunteers trained and supervised by a certified chaplain.[7] Certainly, there was a strong volunteer corps at Glengrove, but they were involved mainly with helping in the deli and gift shop and with running bingo—as well as raising substantial funds for Glengrove. Whether they would be willing to take part in a far more intensive role of listening and sharing with those in pain from illness or death was another matter.

The role of the chaplain was particularly important at Glengrove because it didn't have a full-time social worker for the ALF residents. Susan, the manager of the residential units, was a social worker, but her primary responsibilities centered on managing the apartments. Glengrove had a social worker housed in its nursing home section, but she seldom visited the residents. Her primary tasks related to completing government forms for payments to the nursing home. ALF residents who encountered problems could not readily draw on her skills as a social worker.

SPEAKING WITH MOTHER: STAYING IN TOUCH

The telephone was my primary means for staying in touch with my mother. I telephoned her at least twice each week, and she called me as often. She was generally in an up mood, though sometimes concerns or depression were evident. She also had a network of younger friends and family who telephoned and visited. I estimated that about three times each month there were visitors with whom she dined or shopped—sometimes introducing them to restaurants she had discovered.

My mother continued to visit Barbara, my brother's widow, and Barbara's mother, Rita. Both were observant Christians. When my brother died, Barbara's father, who died about a year later, promised that his family would include my mother as part of their family. My mother always was part of their Christmas celebrations; these began Christmas morning with a giant breakfast, held on the first floor of the large, old home of one of Barbara's brothers, a meal everyone, including my mother, helped to prepare. The celebration then moved upstairs, where an apartment had been built for Rita when her husband became ill. My mother reached the second floor on a moving chair, which she found an exciting ride, made safe by Barbara walking at her side.

The Christmas tree and gifts followed, along with two other meals, properly spaced. Barbara was always ready to bring my mother back to Glengrove by early afternoon, if she wished. Until the year she died, however, my mother preferred to stay until the festivities were over, at about 8 p.m.

At Thanksgiving, Glengrove had dinners for residents and nursing home patients in the cultural center with, as my mother said, "all the trimmings." And at Passover, Rabbi Nathan ran the somewhat abridged seders, which lasted only a few hours. Sometimes my mother chose to spend Thanksgiving and Passover with my cousin Mel and his wife, Irene. At Passover, enjoying the best of both worlds, she attended the second night seder at Glengrove.

My mother continued to visit me in Toronto twice each year. The airline staff telephoned to remind her of the flight and to make sure she had received the tickets. They also helped with the wheelchair that made it easier for her to carry the cartons of strudel and cookies she had prepared for me.

I noticed that as long as my mother didn't have to climb stairs, she could easily take short walks, which we enjoyed together. Yet, one of her greatest pleasures in her visits was being able to take long and leisurely baths, something she was unable to do at Glengrove with its shower-only amenities.

The visits and the traditions began to tail off for my mother in the third year of her residence at Glengrove, when she had the first of several falls. Until that time, it is fair to say that, as a consumer, my mother (like most ALF residents) would have considered herself highly satisfied with her life at Glengrove. I think she would have disagreed strongly with Jacquelyn Frank, an anthropologist and professor at Illinois State University, who wrote that, despite the "high-satisfaction" scores, researchers didn't observe much joy among the ALF residents: "For $5,000 a month, I'd sure like to hear someone say, 'I'm having a good time. I'm enjoying my life.' Not just, 'It's not as bad as it could be. It's not as bad as a nursing home.' That's sad."[8]

In spite of my mother's satisfaction with her early years at Glengrove, I became convinced that, in an instant, she, like most ALF residents, would give up tenancy happily—given a choice, given the opportunity to turn back the clock, to be healthy, to live in the company of old friends, with family. But, they knew that the choice was not theirs to make. They could only hope to find some level of satisfaction in the reality they faced.

4 The Staff and the Boss

SECURITY

Months before she moved to Glengrove, my mother told me she had been awakened late at night by someone pounding on her front door. Through the curtains she had seen three young men, one holding a whiskey bottle, all laughing. She called the police, but by the time they arrived the men had left. From neighbors, she learned they were looking for a party and had the wrong address. Still, she had been frightened.

Her security was a concern for her and for me. She expected Glengrove to have adequate security staff to ensure her safety and the protection of her property. But doubts soon arose. During the early months of her stay, my visits were frequent, and we often went out to dinner with relatives or friends. When we returned to Glengrove, usually at about nine o'clock, we always found the entrance locked. No one was in the front office near the door. There was only an audio-intercom button, answered by staff in the nursing home section of the facility, which was far from the apartments.

Without identifying herself, my mother would tell the voice at the other end that she wanted to go to her apartment. The voice asked for no identification, and my mother then was admitted. No one later checked her apartment to ensure that she was the person they had buzzed in.

"You know," my mother said to me, "in your apartment building in Toronto there are security people at a desk when you come in, and there are security people in the corridors leading to the apartments. Why shouldn't we have the same kind of protection here?"

My mother, Alice, and other residents thought this lack of an evening attendant was wrong. They felt this was too important a matter to simply accept. Seeking help, they spoke not with Glengrove's management but with their adult children. They did not use the residents' association to voice a grievance, but through their adult children word of their concern reached the administration. Weeks later, an attendant was placed in the office adjacent to the apartment entrance during the night shift.

The job of the attendant was to check on late arrivals and departures. This was not easy since the attendant, from Eastern Europe, appeared to have difficulty understanding either the residents or their guests. She seemed to rely on visual clues, but even that was difficult because she sat in an enclosed office adjacent to the door and had to shout to be heard by anyone passing her.

Mediocre security is not an uncommon problem at ALFs. Many promise a secure environment but don't seem to spend the money to keep that promise. At one ALF in St. Paul, Minnesota, a resident had a medical emergency to which no one responded because they didn't understand English and couldn't comprehend the cries for help. When the case was investigated, the facility was accused of consumer fraud for promising to have "professionally trained staff" on the premises twenty-four hours a day. What the case illustrated is how broadly some ALFs define the terms "professional" and "trained."[1]

Glengrove had the technology and sometimes the staff to handle many nighttime emergencies. During my mother's stay, there were fire alarms, tornado alerts, and individual calls for help through use of emergency cords in all apartments. A full sprinkler system was in place, as required by state law. These emergencies seemed to have been met efficiently by nursing home staff, who ran down the connecting corridors and arrived at the apartments within five to ten minutes after the alarms went off. Glengrove's nursing home staff was kept at an acceptable level in accord with state law.

There were two fundamental obstacles to the provision of services and security to the residents of Glengrove: the quality of its staff and the resistance of residents to help. By far the largest number of health care workers in the facility, as in all ALFs, were aides. They were the first line in meeting emergencies and, probably more important, in providing preventive health care. Although the job is considered unskilled, the reality was that the job tasks, if properly performed, required significant skills. Aides were told at the time of employment that they were working in an assisted living facility, not a nursing home. This meant that they were to act in ways that encouraged resident independence. For example, residents coping with dementia or impaired physical functions were to be treated patiently and as adults—a distinction most aides apparently understood. What many did not seem to understand was the reality of the normal aging process.

As an influential study of ALFs found, "Most staff . . . had no clear picture of normal aging. The vast majority (i.e., more than three-quarters) thought, for example, that incontinence, confusion, and depression were a normal part of aging, rather than potentially reversible conditions that could be the result of some treatable disease process or physiological problem."[2] Unfortunately, better-trained staff such as licensed practical nurses and registered nurses are in short supply in most ALFs. LPNs who work in such facilities often monitor ten or more residents. One-third of ALFs have no RN on staff.

Aides therefore provide much of the hands-on resident care in facilities like Glengrove. Yet, according to the study, one-quarter of the ALFs studied had only one aide for each twenty-three or more residents. Glengrove seemed no different. From 8 a.m. to 4 p.m. there were health care aides in abundance on the apartment floors of Glengrove. Susan said there was probably one aide for every ten to thirteen residents. "Probably" seemed to be the operative term because, depending on the day and the staff turnover, the ratio of aides to residents might be lower.

Aides at Glengrove, as at other ALFs, had to deliver meals, do laundry and housekeeping, and deal with residents who may have significant problems with mobility and other activities of daily living (ADL). "[The data quoted raise] questions about whether such ALFs could allow significant aging-in-place and meet the needs of residents with even moderate ADL impairment," the study concluded.[3]

In 2000 there were 1.26 million aides in the United States. By 2030, individuals over sixty-five will make up 20 percent of the U.S. population. The demand for aides has increased. Estimates are that by 2011 there will be a need for six hundred thousand more of these direct caregivers. Their occupation is now among the top ten in the United States, with the fastest job growth rate. But their pay has remained low. In 2000 their national average was $7.56 an hour. This compared to wages for retail sales of $8.64 and factory work at $10.30 an hour. As a report sponsored by the assisted living industry further explained, "Unfortunately, long-term care has traditionally been an unattractive field in which to work. The work is physically and emotionally demanding, the hours are long, the wages are low compared to the work required and, unfortunately, many facilities have not offered benefits in the past."[4]

Aides usually lack experience, training, and certainly any specialized certification for their job. The orientation or training they receive tends to be on the job and generally is limited to no more than seventy-five hours. Depending on the nature of that training, it is possible for it to lead to job promotion as "assistant nurse." This category does not exist at many ALFs and is not related to the certification and licensing of registered nursing assistants (RNAs). Rather, it is a small promotion with some additional compensation reflecting enhanced job skills.

With a few exceptions, the job of aide is a dead end. Without significantly more education and without certification, the aide cannot expect to enter the next compensation level of health care. Most of those jobs are in nursing homes. Even if the aide finds the means to qualify for some certification, job openings will be limited. ALFs employ few nurses or other professionals (e.g., physical therapists).

Because of this, turnover among aides in the long-term care industry is high. In 2000 the annual national rate of aide turnover reported by the Assisted Living Federation of America was 93 percent. This was seen as a sign that "we as an industry are slowly making changes necessary in order to keep our quality workers." According to that report, the national average turnover in 1995 was 106 percent.[5] Another study echoed that finding in its estimate that 20 percent of aides had been on the job less than six months. According to the same study, aide turnover rates in different facilities ranged up to 200 percent.[6]

No employee turnover statistics were made available to residents or their families at Glengrove. There was only the sense that aides came and went with great regularity. However, in work scheduling, Glengrove, like most high-service ALFs, did attempt to have aides responsible to the same residents. On occasion, my mother thought she saw former aides employed as servers at the riverboat casino she frequented for its buffet and twenty-five-cent slot machines.

Glengrove initiated its own low-cost program to keep employees. For those who were on the job for three years, a small "appreciation" raise was awarded, along with a "loyalty" pin. (Glengrove's activities director proudly showed me her pin.)

Staff turnover at Glengrove became a concern to me. Safety, after all, was an important reason that I urged my mother to consider moving there. When she was living alone, I had pictured her falling down the steep cellar stairs when doing her laundry or from a stepladder while painting or cleaning walls, with no one there to help her.

I saw Glengrove as a place where such risks were minimal. I

imagined that there was a staff member always available to help. If my mother fell in her apartment, she needed only to pull a nearby cord for help. If she didn't appear for an expected function (such as dining), then staff would enter her apartment to ensure she was all right. Indeed, from time to time, an aide would enter her apartment just to make sure everything was okay.

Both my mother and I were willing to accept a trade-off: having the safety we wanted meant that not just one but a number of persons had keys to my mother's apartment. These included the aides, the front office (including the LPN and Glengrove's manager), and the dining room manager. We were willing to accept that the privacy that she had in her home was at an end.

During my mother's early years at Glengrove, she and I differed on how we viewed the role of aides. Just as she had resisted help from the geriatric nurse I had called to evaluate the safety of her house, she often viewed the presence of aides as an unwanted ALF judgment of her growing dependence on others. Initially, she thought of the aides—who were all female—as housekeeping staff. They were there to tidy up her apartment or to do a bit of laundry. Often, my mother never got to know their names because they didn't seem to stay very long on the job.

Generally, at about 8 a.m., an aide knocked on her door. Most of the time, she was up and functioning. The aide would enter and vacuum the floors lightly, dust, and put a few dishes in the dishwasher. If there was any laundry, she did it. (The cost was added to the monthly rent.)

My mother knew that the aide did other things, but she didn't think much about what those things were. Her friend Alice, who was in full possession of her senses, had a somewhat different view. Alice wanted to get dressed quickly and needed some help. On most mornings, the aide who came to vacuum Alice's apartment also made her bed and helped her dress. The aide checked a box on a work ticket marked "dressing assistance," which she turned in to her supervisor at the end of her shift. This became an add-on to Alice's monthly rental.

My mother was aware that aides helped Alice dress. But she

certainly didn't want that kind of service for herself—at least during the first three years she lived at Glengrove. She wanted to be independent and didn't want aides to clean her apartment. "I can do a better job in half the time," she said. If anything, she wanted the aides to be invisible. But when her own capacities diminished, she, like Alice, became more accepting of help. Even then, however, she showed a certain annoyance toward aides, which I thought came from her own frustration at not being able to do all those things that marked her independence.

On request, aides also helped those residents using walkers or wheelchairs to move within the facility. Such help often was given when a resident was new to the use of a walker or wheelchair. This assistance also became a ticketed item for which Glengrove, like other ALFs, imposed an additional charge termed "employee assisted in-house transportation." It carried a fee of $40 a month.

Rather than viewing the aides as part of a much-needed security system, my mother's main concern seemed to be to limit the access of aides to her apartment. She did not want anyone uninvited to enter her home. This was a privilege reserved for friends, family, and workers hired to do a specific job. She was content to have someone come every day to do the kinds of chores aides do. What she had difficulty handling was that the aides themselves were always changing, always strangers. She had limited privacy. As one study stated,

> As in most residential care settings, staff turnover in assisted living is a major concern. In focus group interviews, both resident and family members cited low staff turnover as a key indicator of quality. . . . Stability among staff offers the opportunity for more consistent care and a staff that is more familiar with and attuned to individual resident needs and preferences. In assisted living, as in other such settings, personal care assistants or aides have the highest turnover rates among all direct care staff members.[7]

My mother and other residents were also concerned that aides might be spying on them and reporting back to management. In fact, though aides were not spying, they did play an important monitoring role—part of the trade-off between privacy and security.

Some aides at Glengrove with significant seniority developed close relationships with residents. But at times they felt conflicted. They were expected to report any apparent problems regarding a resident's ability to live safely and "properly" in her apartment. This included reporting excessive dirtiness in the apartment, signs of incontinence (such as stained floors or bed linen), and food spoilage. As well, aides were to report unusual behavior.

An aide was expected just to observe—but not discuss what she observed with the resident or her family. At Glengrove reports (usually verbal) were made to Susan, or whoever was the resident manager at the time. Susan then visited the tenant in her apartment. It was styled a casual visit, but its purpose and end result might be serious, assuming the aide's report was accurate. It could, using incontinence as an example, even lead to a resident's "de-admission." In effect, the aides acted as a surveillance force for Glengrove's management.

It was only in my mother's last years at Glengrove that, by chance, I became aware of how problematic this surveillance could be. I was visiting her, and, as had been my custom, I stopped first at the office to say hello and see if there were any problems. By then, Susan had been temporarily replaced as residence manager by Teresa, a woman in her thirties with a business degree specializing in management and a limited command of English. This was her first job in the United States. Before she came to Glengrove, she had worked as a bureaucrat for an Eastern European government agency. With her fixed smile, she broadcast the attitude of technocrat. The first time I saw her, she was in the process of berating Sally, a newly employed aide in her twenties.

Teresa asked Sally why she had not reported that my mother had shown signs of incontinence. She demanded a full report.

Sally falteringly replied that she hoped my mother would be okay. That, Teresa said, wouldn't do. "You were instructed when you were first employed that I am to be told immediately when any resident shows signs of not being able to care for herself."

Then Teresa looked up and saw me at the door. She told Sally to leave and welcomed me. Wearing that same fixed smile, Teresa assured me that she would speak with my mother. How, I asked, did she intend to speak with my mother? "Quite directly," Teresa answered. "She knows our rules. But please understand that I will be polite."

Bee, one of the LPNs on staff, heard the entire conversation. (Their offices were adjacent and the doors were open.) One of the few veterans at Glengrove and a friend of my mother, Bee bustled into the room and said, "Let me speak to his mother. I know how to do it in a way that won't offend her. We can start her on pads. And she will know that lots of other residents have the same problem." This was how I learned about my mother's incontinence and how it would be handled the first time.

THEFT AND THE LOCKED DRAWER

It was the second day of a visit with my mother. The previous evening, she and I had gone out for ribs, her favorite dinner. She seemed quite happy, and the conversation was light. The following morning, I arrived at her apartment to pick her up for breakfast with Barbara and her mother.

Alice and my mother—whose faces were serious, even glum— met me at the door. Alice took the lead: "We didn't want to worry you on your visit. But your mother and I talked it over, and we both feel you simply have to know. In the last few weeks, we have had things taken. We are both missing money, and your mother's special broach is gone. We don't know for sure who did it, but we suspect it was Diane, the new aide. It's only a suspicion. But both of us have seen her opening dresser drawers in our apartments. She said it was only to arrange some linens—and there were linens in both drawers."

Alice and my mother wanted to know what to do. Theft, they said, was a problem common to Glengrove. Alice wanted her money back. She wanted an end to thefts. She wanted to feel comfortable leaving her cash on a table or jewelry in a drawer. "It wasn't as if either your mother or I left thousands or even hundreds of dollars out," she said. "We don't have that kind of money. And it wasn't as if your mother's jewelry was valuable— except in her eyes. But this is our home. We're forbidden from putting extra locks on the door. We have to let the aides and others into our apartments. We're not living in a hotel where guests are put on notice of possible thefts and advised to take their valuables with them or put them in a safe." (In fact, Glengrove did have a safe where residents could check valuables.)

The only choice, according to Alice and my mother, was not to have anything that might invite theft. I said that I understood their concerns and that I would look into the matter.

My first stop, after breakfast, was a visit with Susan. She listened (as she always did). Then she told me how things stood. Except when an employee was actually caught stealing, there was little Glengrove could do. When I asked why, Susan asked me to consider the difficulties. How could you prove that something had been taken? Who was to be charged with the theft? How could that person's guilt be proved? If all these questions were answered, then what was the remedy? Who would impose it? And how could the problem of theft be prevented?

Susan left no doubt that theft from residents was a problem. She readily acknowledged that a number of employees had keys to apartments and that this was for the residents' protection. At least, Susan said, apartment residents had locks on their doors. There were no locks on the doors in the nursing home. Anyone—other residents, employees, visitors—could enter a room. Valuables—indeed, anything of interest—left in view could be taken. The fact that Glengrove had a safe where residents and patients could store their valuables had little practical meaning. The objects or cash taken from Alice and my mother were intended to be used, not stored in a safe.

When my mother died in Glengrove's nursing home, I learned the truth of Susan's comment about the absence of locks there. Taken from her room within forty-eight hours of her death were a special doll, which she had named after her mother, and a vase filled with silk flowers, given to her as a present and greatly prized. I reported the theft to the head nurse, who took careful notes. And that was the last I heard of the matter.

Theft is an endemic problem at both high-end and low-end ALFs and nursing homes. In its hiring program, Glengrove did attempt to control employee wrongdoing. There might have been limited orientation for aides, Susan said, but values and rules were emphasized: Employees have a special relationship with residents, one of trust and caring. The dignity of residents is to be respected, and their independence is to be nurtured. If you violate that trust, your employment is terminated. Further, all employees—aides included—went through a police check. The information obtained was used to filter applicants whose backgrounds gave rise to any risk of potential harm to residents.

I later reviewed these points with Alice and my mother. Alice laughed sarcastically: "These protections, if they can be called that, are okay. But the best kind of protection, from my point of view, would be if, in the contract of admission, Glengrove promised to compensate residents for theft. But there's no way management here would undertake such liability." Alice was right. The contract of admission, for the most part, was not one that could be negotiated.

To catch a thief is no easy matter. The first and most obvious difficulty lies with the victim herself. A resident has to report the theft of, say, a certain sum of money or a specific piece of jewelry. She has to recall approximately when the theft occurred. Often she has to be willing to speak about these matters to a third party, someone unknown to her. And sometimes she has to tell her story in a courtroom-like setting, such as a special hearing where an accused employee, through her union, contests a penalty imposed by management.

None of this is easy for people who feel vulnerable. And it could be very confusing and disorienting to the high percentage of ALF residents who have mild to moderate "cognitive impairment," which often takes the form of forgetfulness or confusion from confrontation.[8]

For my mother and Alice there might have been another approach, though it too would have presented difficulties. The aide on duty at the relevant time could be charged not with theft but with opening the dresser drawers of a resident without her permission—assuming that the resident had no cognitive impairment. Alice and my mother would only have had to fix the time when this happened and identify the aide involved.

But how would such a charge be handled, and what effect might it have on the aide and other Glengrove employees? The starting point is the fact that the employees of Glengrove, at least when my mother first lived there, were members of a union, which management had recognized. The union and Glengrove had entered into a contract, binding in law, called a collective agreement, which set the hours, terms, and conditions of employment for those represented by the union.

Among the terms, and common to such agreements, are provisions requiring management to have "just cause" before any employee can be disciplined. The burden of proof is on management not only to show just cause but also to demonstrate that the discipline imposed is appropriate. And this means, for the most part, that the discipline is progressive—except in cases of a fundamental breach of the employee-employer relationship. The employee is put on notice that her actions are wrong and that if they are repeated, a more severe penalty may be imposed, including suspension and even discharge.

My mother and Alice had spoken with Susan. They did not have the power under the collective agreement to seek discipline against any employee. Only the management of Glengrove had that power. For the most part, complaint proceedings against an individual employee, in the form of an arbitration before an independent third party acceptable to the union and management, are not something that either the union or management wants. It is costly, it strains labor relations between the parties, and it can create tension between the residents and the staff.

Susan could have taken another approach. Under a collective agreement, management has the right to set working conditions, except to the extent that the agreement specifically provides otherwise. Susan could have set a rule, posted for employees and residents to see, that stated:

1. The resident's personal effects are not to be touched by employees except with the specific consent of the individual resident.
2. In no case is an employee to open any drawer in a resident's apartment. Residents are urged to report any violation of this rule as soon as it happens. Employees are cautioned that any violation of this rule can lead to discipline, including the possibility of discharge.

For reasons known best to her and Glengrove, no such approach was taken. For that matter, so far as I could determine, no employee code of conduct as to resident property was ever set out. It is a given that theft of a resident's property, a criminal offense, could result in discharge—even in the absence of a management rule.

It might have been that Glengrove had another perspective, one that directly touched its own profit center. The union could have been seen as a threat. The employees accepted the union, at a dues cost to them of about ten dollars monthly. They did this in the hope of better working conditions and better pay, both of which would have proved costly to Glengrove. In the final result, the approach of Glengrove was to marginalize the union, to keep working conditions and pay essentially at the same level as before the union arrived on the scene, and to contract out work where possible—all with the view that employees would, as they did, ask themselves whether they were getting any real benefit from the dues being paid.

Neither a rule nor possible individual action against an individual aide met the concerns of Alice and my mother. Taking matters into their own hands, they approached George, a retired plumber in his sixties employed by Glengrove as a maintenance person. George was a friendly man who was always open for a chat with residents over a cup of coffee and a cookie. My mother and Alice told George of their concerns, suggested a possible solution, and asked if he would help.

Glengrove had a rule, well-known to the residents, which stated that there were to be no locks anywhere in an apartment. But in each apartment bathroom there was a vanity with a deep drawer. My mother and Alice asked George to install locks on their vanity drawers. They could place valuables there in a safe of their own, for which they would have a key and access whenever they wanted. So one day after work, for a small fee covering the cost of the hardware, George installed the locks.

On my next visit, my mother and Alice delighted in showing me the result of their strike for privacy. They said nothing to other residents or to Susan. Aides coming into their apartments might have noticed the locks, but they apparently said nothing. As for their breach of Glengrove's no-lock rule, my mother simply said, "What they don't know won't hurt them."

When, as my mother approached death and her apartment was given up, I had to remove its contents, I found the key to the locked drawer and I opened it. There were no valuables, only cosmetics—including lipstick, which I had never seen her wear. Hidden under clothing in dresser drawers, I found small envelopes from the Glengrove's branch bank containing a few dollars each. All of her antique costume jewelry was gone.

THE ADMINISTRATORS AND THE BOSS

Susan, Bee, Cindy, and Anne—Glengrove manager, LPN, activities director, and manager of the dining room, respectively—along with Sylvia, head of volunteers, were the human face of Glengrove. For the most part, they were the staff with whom my mother came into daily contact. My expectation, and that of my mother, was that they would be there for the long term. I assumed that they were people my mother would grow to know and view as a kind of extended family. But this became difficult. Here too there was high staff turnover, sometimes due to what seemed to be ever-changing operational responsibilities, and sometimes simply because people were searching for a better work life.

During my mother's tenancy, the position of apartment manager changed four times. Susan, a senior employee and social worker, had first interviewed my mother at Glengrove. There was an immediate bond between the two. My mother often began her daily stroll around Glengrove with a visit with Susan—a visit that Susan seemed to enjoy.

About a year after my mother came to Glengrove, Susan was transferred when she was given the operational responsibility for setting up and marketing the former Alzheimer's and dementia wing that had been converted to small rental units. Susan was thought to be the person with the experience and skill to best market these. Susan's transfer occurred without notice and without discussion. One day Susan was in her office at Glengrove. The next day, when my mother came to visit, she was gone. And although Susan tried to stay in touch with my mother and some other residents, she had little time. Her new job involved going into the community to explain and market the new units. When she wasn't speaking before a community group, she was interviewing applicants and helping them to get settled.

Two other managers were later installed in what had been

Susan's office. Again there was no notice, no discussion with residents, no introductions. Just a new face behind a desk, the office door closed more often than not. If there was any master plan in their placement, it may have been to groom them for later positioning in the nursing home or in the administration of the facility.

In the fourth year of my mother's stay, Susan—again without announcement or discussion with residents—was returned to the apartments. This time, however, she had a double responsibility. She was to manage both the apartments and the low-cost units, which had been fully rented through her efforts. How Susan was to manage both parts of the ALF, physically distant from each other, was another matter. What Glengrove got was one supervisor doing the job of two—and being paid slightly more than she had earned before.

Susan was stressed. She once told me that she had considered quitting, but her loyalty to the institution, as she put it, kept her there. Her office phone, cell phone, and pager were constantly ringing. The only way to reach her was by leaving a voice message. She did return calls.

Residents benefited from Susan's presence when she was available. But the relationship between the residents, their family members, and Susan clearly was not as intimate as it had been in the first year.

My mother and other residents quickly became attached to Cindy, the activities director, who was outgoing, warm, and seemed to be quite willing to expand her normal forty-hour week to fit their needs and desires. At the end of the first year, Cindy resigned to take a similar position with another ALF, which, she said, was closer to her home.

Word of her leaving came in a chance comment that Cindy made to me on one of my visits. Residents learned through Glengrove's grapevine. If they had been given the chance, residents and family members could have discussed with Cindy to see what, if anything, might have induced her to stay. And at the very least, they would have given Cindy a good-bye party. But Cindy turned in her resignation, which management accepted.

Marsha, Cindy's successor, and the residents had some difficulty adjusting to each other. This was no small matter, for activities formed a central part of daily life at Glengrove. It would not do for residents to sulk and refuse to go on outings because Marsha wasn't Cindy. In the end, however, the transition seemed to work out. Marsha stayed on, and after three years she was awarded a gold pin for her length of service—recognition she clearly valued.

Who, I wondered, made the decisions to assign and reassign Susan, and to simply accept Cindy's resignation? The answer, I assumed, was the chief executive officer of Glengrove. Yet, the reality was that that office, like the aide and line management, also was subject to significant turnover.

In Glengrove's first six years there were four CEOs. The first served in a transitional role, the second retired, and the third died following surgery. The fourth was selected after an executive search. I overheard a candidate for the CEO's job being coached by a headhunter in a Glengrove hallway before his interview. "Remember," she said, "to tell them you're a team player." I don't know whether that candidate got the job. The CEO tenure at Glengrove was less than the ALF industry's median length of service of 2.5 years.

I do know that the residents were not consulted with regard to any of the CEOs, nor were their families. The CEO did attend residents' association meetings. At no point, however, did any newly installed CEO speak with the residents about his vision for Glengrove or, more important, sound out the residents to learn how they wanted to see Glengrove function.

One can question the skills that ALF administrators bring to their jobs. A study found that more than four-fifths of them had worked in the health care sector before assuming their current position, but almost a quarter had received no training in operating a facility for the frail elderly. The highest educational level of administrators, reached by less than one-third of those questioned, was a bachelor's degree. About a quarter had some post-baccalaureate education.[9]

The Glengrove CEOs were, in fact, administrators acting under supervision—not from the board of directors but from the longtime chair of the board, Emily Hahn. She was the person who really shaped the residents' experiences through her financial management strategies, which had a great social and financial impact not just on residents but on their families.

Mrs. Hahn, in her sixties, was the head of a wealthy Jewish family. While her husband was still alive, she took a major role in managing the privately held family manufacturing business. When her husband died, she assumed full control.

She was highly intelligent and enormously energetic. For decades, her family had contributed heavily to community and religious charities. But Mrs. Hahn had long had the desire to "adopt" a charity, one on which she could put her own stamp and ensure that it ran effectively and met its defined goals. The charity she selected to adopt was Glengrove. Her approach was to make major contributions, totaling in the millions, for two wings in Glengrove that bear her family name.

Whatever her "regular" business duties, she always had time for Glengrove. On most days and especially on weekends, she visited residents, talked with staff, and made her presence felt. Both residents and staff understood that they were talking with "a very important person." At least three times each year, at her own expense, she brought residents from Glengrove to her family "ranch in the city." There, urban cowhands put on a small rodeo, and residents were taken for safe and secure, but for them exciting, pony rides, followed by a western barbecue.

From her point of view, to be successful an ALF—charitable or for-profit—had to be operated on a solid and stable financial basis. She believed that Glengrove's business plan, from the start, was flawed. To stay in the black, the plan assumed that nursing home beds would be filled. This would have assured a steady flow of government dollars sufficient for the nursing home, and it even would have generated a small surplus for added activities.

For a number of reasons, not the least of which related to changes in government funding cutbacks, Glengrove's nursing home had a large number of bed vacancies during the first few years of operations. To achieve the bottom line Mrs. Hahn decided it was necessary to substantially increase rents and related charges, such as medication administration, to the ALF residents.

Mrs. Hahn could have gone to the Jewish community that had contributed heavily toward funding the construction of Glengrove and had continued funding programs. To Mrs. Hahn, however, this was not enough. Each time Glengrove had financial difficulties, she did not want to go "hat in hand" and seek additional funding from other charities.

Her vision for Glengrove was that it "should be run like a business," a corporate goal she put to her board of directors. Some directors, longtime supporters of Glengrove, rejected the proposal. Their response was that the operation of Glengrove was not a business but a charitable endeavor long supported by the Jewish community.

Mrs. Hahn answered that if Glengrove were run like a business, it would not be necessary to ask for increased contributions. And after all, she stated, the best kind of charity is when one does not have to ask for it. The board listened, raised some questions, and finally a majority allowed Mrs. Hahn to develop and implement a new business plan.

The board, for the most part, consisted of laypersons whose primary interests were outside Glengrove. They cared about the welfare of the institution, but they were uninterested in spending any more time on it than an interested volunteer might. They would be happy if the eager and committed Mrs. Hahn would use her business savvy to rescue Glengrove. Mrs. Hahn, in effect, became the boss.

Her calculus apparently included a steady increase in rents and fees designed to place Glengrove within the high-cost end for ALFs, an end that would still bring full apartment occupancy based on a quality reputation. A majority of Glengrove's board did not challenge the results of her policy.

In the first year of my mother's tenancy, residents and their families were informed of a rent increase of 15 percent—far in excess of the rate of inflation. The justification offered in a brief letter from the chief executive officer was that the increase was necessary because of inflationary pressures. There was no meaningful opportunity for discussion by residents or their children.

And there seemed no choice for the residents, or their adult children, but to pay the increase. For several days, there were hopeful whispers of a rent strike. But that was as far as my mother's generation of seniors would take the matter. To speak loudly might upset the staff. It might even reach the ears of senior management, or "the boss," Mrs. Hahn. The residents seemed fearful of upsetting the management, who they believed might make life unpleasant.

I pause here to note two Canadian stories of resident action that brought broad media coverage. In 2004 Roland Clegg, ninety-two, a retired farmer, was resident with his wife in a thirty-two-room ALF complex run by an agency of the Manitoba government. Without notice to the residents, the agency effectively removed emergency call service cords that had been installed in each resident apartment. The cords were tied to the ceiling.

It was the agency view that the emergency service was being overused. The residents were told that they could purchase a form of med-alert for about forty dollars a month. Many of the residents argued that the price was more than they could afford and that, in any event, the service would be too slow. Moreover, the emergency cord service, they claimed, had been included in their contract of tenancy.

Mr. Clegg led a rent strike. He urged residents to withhold

monthly rent checks until the service cords were restored. Most of the residents signed a declaration that stated: "We are withholding our rent checks pending a thorough investigation of the (management) decision."

Helen Johns, eighty-three, a widow and a resident, took part in the rent strike. "It's pretty scary," she said. "What are they going to do with us? I've never done anything like this in my life, but I don't know what else we can do."

Officials of the government agency agency met with the residents, some of their adult children, and a member of the provincial legislature. In a letter to me, Mr. Clegg wrote: "Yes, we got our pull cords again. It was worth the struggle. [The government was] not happy with our action, but it worked."[10]

In another story, action taken by a single person brought major media coverage. Marie Geddes, eighty-six, a two-year resident in a long-term care facility run by the Alberta government, began a hunger strike over the lack of adequate staff. She said that there were only two aides to care for seventeen residents. Ms. Geddes, a diabetic, said, "I decided this was the only way I was going to get help. . . . Many of the patients can no longer speak for themselves. . . . But I can. . . . I waited forty-five minutes on the toilet this morning for someone to come. You wait and wait and they're too busy to come put me to bed." Her concern was raised in the Alberta legislature.[11]

I have noted these stories to illustrate that it is possible for residents and their adult children to speak and be heard. I do not suggest this as a course of action for the purpose of confrontation but rather as a recognition that residents do have a voice, and it is one that should command the respect of ALF management.

But for the most part, that voice is silent, and in its place is fear. For the Glengrove residents this was not an unrealistic fear. After all, they didn't really have the option of leaving. After several months of residence, they tended to be bonded both to other residents and the institution. Moves after that point carry physical and emotional risks. And where else would they go? Other ALFs—particularly for-profit facilities—followed the same kinds of policies and operated under the same imperatives. After moving, things might be even worse. So, many residents simply cut their individual spending, perhaps thinking that it might lighten the financial load on their children.

Glengrove's rent and fee increases were a surprise to me and to many residents and their families. Mrs. Hahn's business model had not been described to us. Further, we knew little of the financial difficulties of the facility. By the last year of my mother's residence at Glengrove, her rent had increased to over three thousand dollars per month—almost twice the amount she had originally paid.

Two and a half years after entering Glengrove, all the money from the sale of my mother's home had been used, and I was paying for her rent and prescription drugs, whose costs were also escalating. For me, the real cost was high. In effect, every dollar paid to Glengrove cost me about two dollars. The reasons: taxes and dollar exchange rates. The money I took from my retirement plans, then tax sheltered, was taxed as ordinary income. And to transfer that money into U.S. dollars was costly, with the Canadian dollar often worth only sixty U.S. cents at that time.

Sometimes, paying my mother's bills promptly became an exercise in black humor created by the policies of bureaucratic institutions like Glengrove and the various banks through which payments were transferred. Bills often would arrive late—not because of any problem with the U.S. or Canadian post offices but because of glitches in computer software.

Canada does not have zip codes of the same type as in the United States. Its postal codes, unlike U.S. zip codes, include letters as well as numbers. Without the proper postal code affixed, the mail inevitably would be slowed. When this happened, I carefully explained to Glengrove's employees and their supervisors how the Canadian postal code differed from that of the

United States. Still, neither Glengrove nor the supplementary insurance company that helped pay my mother's medical bills transcribed the appropriate Canadian postal code.

After several telephone calls to each institution, I received a common answer: "Our computer system is not equipped to input Canadian postal codes." Glengrove indicated that "in several months" new software would be installed that could handle the problem. The supplementary health insurance carrier said there simply was nothing that could be done.

I suggested that the proper postal code could be handwritten on my mother's bill. The answer: "Sorry. The bills go out in block, not individually." I suggested that the bills addressed to me could be faxed or e-mailed. That would allow me to make payment well in advance of any deadline. The answer: "Sorry. That simply is not our policy."

Finally, I called the CEO at Glengrove, who ordered that my mother's bills be directed to him. He then inscribed by hand the appropriate Canadian postal code. Several months later, new software was installed at the facility which allowed for my Canadian postal code to be included in the database.

Dealing with the health insurance company was another matter. Its phone system seemed to be directed by voice mail only. Finding a supervisor with responsibility for mail billing, either by phone or e-mail, seemed impossible. So, I took another approach.

A subbranch of a local bank had opened an office at Glengrove which had limited hours twice weekly. It was staffed by one person, a senior clerk at the bank, Sally, who was mature, approachable, responsible, and quite willing to use her discretion within the limits of her authority. I told Sally about the difficulty in receiving and paying health insurance bills. She agreed to have the bills forwarded to her, and she wrote checks on an account that I had opened for operating expenses. All my mother had to do was fill out the change of address form on her bill. That was done in Sally's presence. The health insurance zip code problem was solved. The means for receiving important bills had been established.

The billing problems were resolved, but the costs kept mounting, and my own retirement plans were put on hold. Upon reflection, I realized that, when my mother's life at Glengrove had begun, I had no clear idea of the overall cost of her stay. I didn't know how long she would live; I didn't know how much rents would escalate; and I certainly couldn't have predicted that the costs would be more than $200,000 Canadian. I never discussed my own financial arrangements with my mother, though my guess is that she was aware—at least in a general way—of what I was doing. My assurances that money was not a problem often were met by measured skepticism, sometimes followed by a roll of her eyes.

While I was able to bear these costs, some residents were not. Rachel was one of them. By the end of her second year at Glengrove, Rachel's savings had been exhausted. Her physical health was good, but she often came to my mother in a depressed state because she did not know what would happen the following year when she would not be able to pay the rent. My mother had no answers.

Rachel brought the problem to Susan, who, as a longtime social worker, knew of possible programs that could provide rent subsidies. And she knew the social work staff at the local welfare office, located only a few miles away. But Susan did not act either in contacting members of that staff or in providing suggestions to Rachel. Instead, she waited until the accounting department at Glengrove ran out of patience about rent nonpayment, a period of about five months.

Although Susan was concerned about Rachel and other tenants strapped for funds, she was not able to access the kind of government rent subsidy programs that might have helped. To do so I thought would have undercut Mrs. Hahn's financial plan, designed to bring in wealthier residents—or at least residents with wealthy children. Under her plan, Mrs. Hahn appeared to think, she could increase rents and raise charges for related services without risking residents' protests. She knew that welfare programs directly or indirectly demanded accountability and put ceilings on the amount of any subsidy.

Mrs. Hahn's strategy seemed to work. She had needed residents like Rachel to fill units when Glengrove opened. But there was a lengthy waiting list for apartments by the end of Glengrove's second year of operation. Rachel was no longer needed as a resident in the larger one-bedroom apartments. Still, Mrs. Hahn was sensitive to Rachel's problems and those of other residents similarly situated. The solution suggested to Rachel, and others under similar financial pressure, was accommodation in the then new smaller residential units called the Gardens.

Units in the Gardens, as we saw, were opened after residents with Alzheimer's or severe dementia were moved to upper-level wards. These self-contained units, each with its own washroom/shower and mini kitchenette, were considerably smaller than a one-bedroom apartment. But the units had locks on the door and a sense of privacy similar to that of the apartments.

With only her Social Security and her monthly pension, Rachel seized the opportunity to end her financial worries, even though it meant being able to keep only a small part of her belongings. The rest was given to Glengrove's volunteers for auction.

I saw Rachel several months after her move. Probably because of the considerable distance between the Gardens and Glengrove's apartments (or perhaps because of the apartment residents' elitism), she had lost the social circle she had built in the apartment complex. Her friends seemed to be limited to other residents of the Gardens.

Rachel invited me to look at her new apartment. It contained a bed, a small table, two chairs, a sink, and a microwave. There was a small washroom with a shower. A few pictures hung on the walls. Rachel, however, was in good spirits. She said her new dwelling was "cozier" than her one-bedroom apartment, and the residents of the Gardens were friendlier than those in the apartments.

A year after Rachel moved to the Gardens, her rent, along with that of other residents, was substantially increased. Again, she was faced with financial pressure. She could no longer afford the rent of her Gardens apartment, which had been funded from her Social Security payments and a small pension. Glengrove found another place for her—space in the nursing home.

At this point Rachel did not need the nursing home, but she felt that she was lucky. She was given a room to herself, and even her own bathroom with a shower. But she now lived in a room with no lock on the door, and her neighbors often were physically and cognitively impaired. Once again, she had to shed possessions, and was reduced to one chair, a few pictures, and Glengrove's institutional bed and dresser. She wasn't allowed a hot plate. All meals, snacks, and drinks had to be taken either in the dining room of the nursing home or the deli.

For this privilege, Rachel signed over her Social Security payments and those of her pension to Glengrove. She was given a small allowance. She no longer had to worry about payment for room and board. Nor did she have to pay for prescription drugs. She was on Medicaid. Effective control over much of her life had been given over to Glengrove. Rachel had followed the financial path from independence to full dependence, from her own apartment to the nursing home. It was not a path that she or other residents of the apartments thought they would follow when they first entered Glengrove.[12]

5 Health

There are those of us who, thanks to genes, lifestyle, or just good luck, will remain physically and mentally vital and alert until the last day of our lives. But for most of us, our capabilities will lessen with the passing years. This doesn't mean, however, that our desire for a decent quality of life will diminish. The life force may remain vital, but it will take a different shape. What my mother wanted for herself was to live out her days as she chose, receiving help when needed.

Unfortunately, Glengrove did not fully embrace an ethic of individual choice that would encourage residents to live in place by helping them to adapt to their changing lives. To honor such a choice involves far more than helping residents put on a sweat suit and encouraging them to do moderate exercises. As Ivan Illich wrote in *Limits to Medicine—Medical Nemesis: The Expropriation of Health*,

> Health designates a process of adaptation. . . . It designates the ability to adapt to changing environments, to growing up and to aging, to healing when damaged, to suffering, and to the peaceful expectation of death. Health embraces the future as well, and therefore includes anguish and the inner resources to live with it. . . .
> A world of optimal and widespread health is obviously a world of minimal and only occasional medical intervention. Healthy people are those who live in healthy homes on a healthy diet in an environment equally fit for birth, growth, work, healing, and dying; they are sus-

tained by a culture that enhances the conscious acceptance of limits to population, of aging, of incomplete recovery and ever-imminent death. Healthy people need minimal bureaucratic interference to mate, give birth, share the human condition, and die.[1]

Any fulfillment of Glengrove's central promise of aging in place depended on how the staff interpreted and negotiated the details. Critical to this process was whether they respected the fact that my mother, like other residents, hoped to stay in her apartment until the end of her life. To her, good health meant limiting medical intervention and institutional meddling so that she could remain in her new home.

My mother could exercise her judgment and limit medical intervention and institutional intrusion only as long as she or I could control events. Of course, I assumed that if there were a real health emergency, Glengrove would promptly call an ambulance and my mother would be taken to the hospital for treatment. I also assumed that once she had recovered, she would immediately return to her apartment for convalescence.

Those assumptions proved wrong with regard to (a) when Glengrove would seek emergency care, (b) how aggressively my mother would be treated, and (c) when she would return to her apartment. I was surprised at the facility's rush to send my mother to the hospital for emergency treatment, shocked at the aggressive treatment, and disturbed that she wasn't permitted to return to her apartment following her hospital stay but instead was sent to the skilled nursing unit, where she became disoriented.

When my mother became more frail, I learned that neither she nor I—her legal proxy—could make decisions regarding her future if our wishes conflicted with the institution's policy—as they often did, especially at the end of her life.

When I visited my mother during her first years at Glengrove, I became aware of the residents' fear that they would not be able to age in place. Susan or someone else in the administration would require them to convalesce in the "sick building." And they knew they might be moved from there to the nursing home. This fear manifested itself in their shying away from residents who had become "incapacitated" and tending not to speak of those who had "passed on." These fears were hardly irrational.

Residents at Glengrove understood Susan's power. As manager of the apartments, she had the authority to start the process that could end their tenancy and shift them into the "sick building." Three of the primary reasons for tenant displacement (apart from inability to pay) were dementia, incontinence, and falls.

Susan, however, was a friend to the residents. She was genuinely committed to the prospect of aging in place. Toward that end, she bent institutional rules in major areas likely to affect residents. I came to look at her as one of the "angels" at Glengrove, though she never saw herself as being especially giving. "After all," she said to me, "we want a place that will properly serve us when we need it." Unfortunately, Susan's ability to intervene was limited.

DEMENTIA

As I said before, my mother used to say that she could remember where a pin dropped a week after it happened. But three years after moving into Glengrove, she began to have frequent memory lapses. This was troubling to both of us because we knew that residents who exhibited signs of dementia—that is, ongoing, substantial forgetfulness—risked displacement. In fact, one study documented that about 27 percent of ALF residents had moderate to severe dementia.[2]

I am convinced that my mother's memory problems were, at least in part, the result of the deep mourning and depression she felt following Alice's death. Alice and my mother were special friends, soul mates who had found each other in old age. They lived their days together. One night, Alice pushed her emergency button. Staff from the nursing home replied with a call to

911. Alice was sent by ambulance to a nearby hospital. Her doctor did not visit her there, claiming that he didn't have privileges at that hospital. My mother received a telephone call from Alice a night after she had been admitted. "It was only gibberish," my mother said. "I couldn't understand her." Alice died the next day. My mother attended the funeral and insisted on going to the burial. Susan accompanied her to both.

My mother did not hide her grief at Alice's death. Aside from being there for her, there was little I could do to soften that grief. No effective chaplaincy infrastructure was in place to provide ongoing help. The rabbi, as I mentioned, held only a part-time position. His time for any resident was limited, though daily prayer services included portions for those in mourning. This was a good but somewhat partial response for my mother's deep grief.

Coping with my mother's increasing forgetfulness became a challenge. I developed my own way of dealing with it. For example, to alert her to a visit from me, I called and asked that she write down when I would arrive. Then I asked her to read the note back to me—simply to confirm what I had said.

One spring day, the first day of a promised visit, I arrived at Glengrove at the time I had indicated. My mother, who was outside with a group of her friends, became agitated when she saw me. She had remembered the day of the visit but, having forgotten to look at the note, she was expecting me several hours earlier. I simply said I was sorry. Thereafter, however, I stopped telling her in advance when I would see her. Each visit became a surprise. This proved exciting for her, and it eliminated a source of agitation for both of us.

When I had dinner with my mother at Glengrove, it was not unusual for her and her dinner companions to repeat stories from their past as often as two or three times in an hour. Not once did anyone say, "You told me that already." They listened as the conversation went into rewind.

Susan could have dealt with such forgetfulness as dementia,

which occurs when the "loss of intellectual functions (such as thinking, remembering, and reasoning)" becomes so severe that it interferes with "a person's daily functioning."[3] At least, she could have referred the resident to her attending physician and the skilled nursing unit to determine whether transfer to the nursing home was needed.

Susan never made such a recommendation. In her view, as many as half of the residents at Glengrove had low to moderate levels of dementia. But she was content to leave them in their apartments so long as they were not a danger to themselves or to others. Her test was not clinical but based on her assessment of the resident's daily living skills. And for all practical purposes, as long as Susan did not ask for a resident to be transferred out of her apartment, that was the end of the matter.

Not once did I hear Susan mention that a resident had Alzheimer's disease, though it accounts for about 70 percent of all dementias for persons older than eighty-five. But what Susan didn't mention, some of the residents' doctors did. Two of them became my mother's attending physicians at different times: Dr. Linda O'Donnell and Dr. Brian Kay. Their diagnosis of "early stage Alzheimer's" took special meaning when my mother was "snared" in the skilled nursing unit, outside the protective shelter Susan provided. There, Susan had no role to play other than being one of a committee that decided whether my mother was fit to return to her apartment.

The doctors had the power to consign my mother not only to the nursing home but to the Rementia unit—that part of the nursing home set aside for Alzheimer's patients. As a result, I often directed my energy to thwarting the attending physicians, a battle my mother simply didn't have the strength to wage.

In part, the impetus for a diagnosis of Alzheimer's came not from my mother's attending physicians but from a hospital emergency room doctor who charted it as a "possibility" when he treated my mother following a fall. It was a "possibility" that doctors at Glengrove turned into a "probability" and later into a reason they would give for her death. That "possibility" took shape in the context of my mother's responses to general questions and her clear disorientation when she was in the hospital. Though they did not order any brain scans or more formal tests, the two attending doctors insisted on clinical grounds that this was the diagnosis, and "Alzheimer's" became the label for her reality.[4]

INCONTINENCE

Memory loss wasn't my mother's only problem. There was also incontinence. I learned about this again when Susan left me a voice mail message in my mother's fourth year at Glengrove: "This isn't an emergency, but I need to speak with you about your mother." Any call from Susan about my mother triggered an emergency reaction in me. For several weeks, Susan said, aides who were cleaning her apartment, doing her laundry, and making her bed had found worsened signs of urinary incontinence. Now, her sheets, mattress, and rug were soiled. Even her clothing, in which she had always taken so much pride, often tended to be soiled. "This can't continue, for reasons of both sanitation and your mother's health," Susan said. "We have to find a way to deal with it. And we have to do so before other residents begin to gossip."

Susan felt that she should talk with my mother and find a solution. I couldn't have been more pleased. I certainly didn't want to talk with my mother about her continued incontinence. Susan made it clear that incontinence was a common problem for the residents. It was, she assured me, a problem that could be handled.

Susan thought that pads should be tried again. They had been tried earlier when the problem first developed but, apparently, were not fully effective. There was a limited supply at Glengrove that Susan could tap. Thereafter my mother would have to purchase them. Susan also thought that my mother needed some help showering, keeping herself well groomed and dressed, and shopping for items she needed such as pads.

Susan thought that this work could be done in about six hours each week. She suggested the services of Margy, a middle-aged woman who contracted with a number of residents to provide companionship or personal services. Margy was not an employee of Glengrove. Arrangements, including billings, would be matters strictly between Margy and me.

In time the cost of this arrangement would become a strain. But the initial and more important concern was to get my mother to accept Margy. Since my mother was sensitive to any increased cost that I had to bear, Margy and I worked out a plan whereby she would simply present herself to my mother and tell her that she would help around the apartment. She would tell my mother that the cost of her services was minimal and that I had already paid for them. It worked. Margy became a kind of companion to my mother, though hardly the friend that Alice had been.

Next there was the matter of the mattress. A new one had to be purchased. "If I tell your mother that a new mattress has to be bought," Susan said, "she will kill me. From her point of view, the mattress she now has is new. She bought it from Alice's son after her death, and frankly, she has something of a sentimental attachment to it."

I suggested what Susan and I called Operation Mattress. We made arrangements with Sylvia, head of Glengrove's volunteers and a friend of my mother, to take her out for lunch at a time when other residents would be engaged in activities away from the residence. I purchased the same kind of mattress that my mother had bought from Alice's family and arranged to have it delivered while she was out. After the old mattress was taken away, Susan would make up the new one. No one, including housekeeping staff, would know what had happened.

Operation Mattress was a success, and my mother never

guessed that she was sleeping on a new mattress. Working together with Susan pleased me because she was always motivated
by the question, What can be done to help the resident stay in
her apartment in relative safety?

So long as my mother was under Susan's care, physicians
were not asked for their input. I, for one, was not convinced
that they would understand or actively support my mother's
goal to live and die in her apartment. Dementia and incontinence are, of course, medical conditions, and a medical diagnosis certainly helps in understanding their cause and prognosis.
But this assumes that a physician has the time to inquire into the
resident's condition, and many of the physicians caring for residents at Glengrove seemed to lack that time.

Later, as a result of research, I learned that many physicians,
as a practical matter, never ask their elderly patients about incontinence. They never ask partly because they don't have the
time and partly because they are poorly prepared to evaluate incontinence—to say nothing about identifying the options available for its proper treatment. The U.S. Centers for Disease Control, reporting on a 1993 study of incontinence in Massachusetts
and Oklahoma, included this partial summary:

> Urinary incontinence (UI)—the involuntary loss of urine sufficient
> to be a problem for the patient or caregivers—affects an estimated 15–
> 30 percent of persons aged greater than or equal to 60 years in the
> United States and is a major cause of admittance to nursing homes. UI
> may be associated with a variety of medical problems such as rashes,
> skin infections, pressure sores, urinary tract infections, and falls, and
> psychosocial problems such as depression, embarrassment, restricted
> social interaction, reduced activities outside the home, reduced sexual
> activity, and sleep disturbances.
>   Despite the dissemination of clinical practice guidelines for UI . . . ,
> many physicians do not know how to diagnose or treat UI. . . . Al-
> though existing therapies can improve two-thirds of UI cases, the find-
> ings in this report suggest that most primary care physicians neither
> routinely ask their elderly patients about UI nor believe they are ade-

quately prepared to evaluate and treat UI. Previous studies have indicated that approximately half of patients with UI reported their physicians had never asked about UI, treated the condition, or referred them for treatment.[5]

Although specialist nurses understand and treat the problem of incontinence in the elderly, neither Glengrove nor many other ALFs provide residents with such specialist services or even refer them to incontinence nurses. Whether incontinence either can or should be treated with medications is not for nonspecialists like me to decide. There are side effects. I am suggesting, however, that greater medical involvement might be helpful in dealing with the problem.

DOCTOR AND PATIENTS

There was an unwritten but well understood rule at Glengrove—as with most ALFs—that resident admission required naming an attending physician to whom the institution could turn should it have any question concerning a resident's health.

Glengrove did not ask for any written medical evaluation of the resident. Based on personal observation and interviews with the resident, Susan decided whether a resident could function independently. Initially, all that Glengrove demanded was a physician's name and telephone number. Determining whether or not the doctor had a clear picture of the resident's condition did not seem to be part of the admission procedure.

A few physicians made regular visits to residents at Glengrove. My mother had two such doctors, Dr. Sol and Dr. Linda. They ordered medications that the ALF obtained. Specially designated health care aides, rather than nurses, usually administered the medications. The attending physicians also ordered regular blood pressure and weight checks, which were charted not so much for personal, on-site perusal as for fax transmission to their offices.

Attending physicians had a most important power over ALF residents: to influence whether and under what conditions they could stay in their apartments or be transferred either to the "sick building" or to the nursing home or its adjacent Rementia unit. It was one matter to allow Susan to decide to accept a resident to Glengrove. Deciding whether that resident later needed skilled care in the "sick building" or the nursing home was, it seemed, an entirely different matter. Doctors recorded their medical judgments about such matters in charts they kept at Glengrove.

Did doctors base their decisions on the residents' quality of life or were they influenced in part on their own wish to avoid malpractice liability? Many doctors who care for the frail elderly seem to believe that a failure to order needed procedures or medications may be risky. At least two of my mother's doctors indicated that should a resident be harmed as a result of such a failure, they might be open to medical malpractice actions and an increase in their already expensive medical malpractice insurance premiums.

As an attorney, I know that most lawyers shy away from taking such cases because the amount of recovery relative to the risk involved is marginal. Most malpractice actions are taken on a contingency-fee basis with the lawyer handling expenses in the hope of a recovery satisfactorily greater than the cost. The likelihood of a high return from a malpractice action involving an elderly resident is not great. But many doctors don't share this view that there is a minimal malpractice risk.[6]

Susan seldom acted against medical judgments. But she did so twice when we collaborated to spring my mother, whom she regarded as a friend, from the sick building and return her to her apartment.

I saw no need to question the role of the doctor when my mother entered Glengrove. Her doctor at the time was Sol, a friend with a good understanding of my mother. This probably was a mistake. I assumed Sol would outlive my mother. He did not. It was also a mistake because neither my mother nor I were aware of a doctor's potential to affect her life at Glengrove. Yet even if we had been aware of that potential, the reality was that we could not have negotiated a different outcome.

Before moving into Glengrove, my mother had limited use for both physicians and hospitals. Aside from giving birth she had never been hospitalized. Nor did she have any significant physician-patient relationship. Her involvement with doctors had been casual, social, and noninvasive. Any tests were taken either in the doctor's office or at the radiology center, a short walk down the hall.

For more than twenty years my mother's doctor had been Walter Gold, the son-in-law of close friends of hers. Walter had made appointments for my mother to see him and personally called to remind her of scheduled visits. He had cautioned her about her weight and high blood pressure and told her to "diet, cut down on salt, and eat more salad." She had followed his instructions—though not when she was invited to those large family dinners at his home.

Walter had a sense of my mother as a person. He knew of her life, her happiness and sadness. He and his family were at her side when my father passed away, just as she was with them when his in-laws died. He could measure her strength and resilience. And if medications ever became necessary, he was in a position to observe their effect on her.

He treated my mother with a full measure of respect—even, on occasion, asking her advice on family matters. He called her "Ida," and she called him "Walter." When he talked with her, there never was even the barest hint of condescension. He treated her with the respect due an older person who had experience, intelligence, humor, and common sense. He knew that she was a healthy person who continued to work around her home even after she retired, and he was aware of her minor medical problems—such as her diminishing eyesight (which she denied).

Walter, previously a healthy person who ran to keep in shape, died of cancer following a long illness. My mother was at his birthday party a few weeks before his death. His parting words to her, which she treasured, were: "You're quite a lady."

My mother missed Walter after he died, but she was willing to accept another doctor. Sol, a university friend who was a general practitioner in her city, was a warm, friendly person who, as I mentioned, was a longtime board member of Glengrove. I told him that I hoped he would be a laid-back doctor who would encourage my mother to live an active life with an absolute minimum amount of medical intervention. Sol was willing to take my mother as a patient. He and I agreed that should any significant medical problem arise, he would let me know so that I could be supportive of her.

My mother's philosophy about doctors did not change as she became older and more frail. Her firmly expressed view was that if she became so ill that her life was in danger, then let the end come in her own apartment. After all, shouldn't aging in place involve dying in place?

Of course, I recognized that Glengrove, like other ALFs, needed to have physician oversight. I knew that my mother would need a physician to take care of medical emergencies—for example, serious injuries such as broken bones resulting from falls—that were not life threatening but required treatment in hospitals. I wanted that treatment option for my mother.

What worried me was that residents' health, as Glengrove defined it, involved a physician's judgment as to whether a resident could continue her independent life in her apartment. Glengrove could compel a resident to have a medical evaluation in the skilled nursing unit. It didn't matter that a resident might object or be able to hire private assistance to stay in her apartment.

I was less worried about this problem when Sol was my mother's attending physician during her first two years at Glengrove. He no longer required visits to his office for checkups; he came to her apartment carrying his small medical case with stethoscope, tongue depressors, and other devices. I think he saw his visits as giving him insight both into how my mother was coping with her new life and into the operations of Glengrove as an institution for which he bore some responsibility as a member of its board of directors. My mother invited him to her birthday parties, and he attended with his wife. My mother and I were saddened when he died of a heart attack.

Soon after Sol's death, Susan reminded me that I needed to find another attending physician. I spoke with my friend Trudy, whose mother had recently entered Glengrove. She had found a doctor who, though young and not a specialist in geriatric medicine, had a good reputation and saw a number of elderly patients. He was willing to take Trudy's mother as a patient—if she were willing to have him as a doctor. The three met. He suggested that Trudy's mother call him Jeff, and he called her Mrs. Namb. She sat near him, Trudy farther back.

He addressed respectful questions to Mrs. Namb, who had just recovered from a complex surgical procedure. She answered and asked several questions of her own, not the least of which was how long the doctor expected her to live. Jeff said she might have several more years of good life. She persisted. Jeff was unruffled. "Will there be another year?" she asked, to which Jeff answered, "For sure." The meeting with Jeff lasted for more than forty-five minutes.[7] He did not rush Mrs. Namb. She asked him to be her attending physician, and he agreed.

There were other meetings between Jeff and Mrs. Namb, which were of the same caliber. I felt good for Trudy and her mother. At least some physicians out there are willing to spend time with elderly patients, respect them, and listen. I telephoned Jeff and asked whether he would see my mother. He answered that he was sorry but he was overloaded with patients.

Neither my mother nor I were as fortunate as Trudy and Mrs. Namb. I found a doctor who specialized in gerontology and had offices close to Glengrove. She was new to her practice. We spoke for about ten minutes on the phone. Yes, she would see my mother, but she wouldn't visit residents at Glengrove; her patients came to her. Her manner was courteous and professional but not warm. My mother agreed to see her. She went to her appointments on Glengrove's bus (for a charge). The arrangement lasted for about four months.

I understand that doctors have to earn a living and that their incomes depend on their ability to see more than a few patients a day. I also know that they aren't paid to sit, listen patiently, and draw an in-depth patient profile. Some physicians tell me that efficiency requires them to identify and deal with specific medical problems swiftly. They also admit that even so, there is an often-unmet need for good physician-patient communications.[8]

My mother and Alice decided on their own to have Dr. Linda as their attending physician. She had, with the blessings of management (through handouts and announcements), opened an office at Glengrove, making use of an examination room the facility provided. A health care aide was in charge of appointments. A large number of residents chose to employ her because she was on the premises, on call, and also available for emergencies during most daylight hours.

Dr. Linda, whom I guessed to be about forty-five, had a smilingly imperious manner with patients. She ordered them about in a peremptory way. There was no cajoling. Though Alice and my mother thought this approach amusing, I wasn't so sure. I first became concerned about Dr. Linda when I learned how she reacted during Alice's last illness and after her death.

After Alice died, my mother did not hide her profound grief. Within Glengrove, her real consolation came from the volunteers. Dr. Linda and Rabbi Benjamin were a constant presence at Glengrove, and since they saw her at activities or at the deli, they had to be aware of her grief. Yet their words of comfort were sparse.

My concerns about Dr. Linda were confirmed during my

mother's first hospitalization and experience with the "sick building." A few months after Alice's death, my mother fell during a grocery shopping trip. She remained conscious and no bones were broken, but the store manager didn't want to take any chances. He called an ambulance, and my mother was taken to the hospital. I was notified by phone. Fortunately Betsy, an alert and very bright niece with common sense, was in town visiting her parents. She volunteered to go to the hospital. Betsy telephoned me from my mother's hospital room, and I was able to speak with my mother. She sounded groggy but lucid. The doctors confirmed that she was in good physical condition and there were only a few bruises. My mother was released to Betsy to be taken back to Glengrove.

Both my mother and Betsy thought that she would return to her apartment. Such, however, was not the policy of Glengrove. Instead my mother was taken to the "sick building," the skilled nursing unit. She was frightened and disoriented, but not too confused to know where she wanted to recover—in her apartment. "Why," she asked, "can't I go back to my home, my apartment?" The nurse in charge of the skilled nursing unit replied, "We want to make sure you will be okay in your apartment. We'll get you back there as soon as possible." Dr. Linda, then available, concurred, and Betsy left.

There was no telephone in the room assigned to my mother. I could not reach Dr. Linda. Later, much later, that evening, I convinced a nurse on my mother's floor to carry a cell phone to her so we could talk. I promised my mother that she would be back in her apartment either the next day or the following day. Dr. Linda disagreed with me, and Susan said that she lacked the power to return my mother to her apartment.

It was Dr. Linda's view that my mother showed signs of Alzheimer's. She was, she said, delusional during the night: She was speaking to my father and my brother, both deceased. She wandered into the room of another patient. She was incontinent and couldn't find the bathroom. "We really ought to keep her here to see whether it might be better for her to be admitted to the nursing home," Dr. Linda announced.

It was at that point that my anger, until then controlled, flared. I quietly but firmly told her that there would be legal consequences if my mother were not returned immediately to her apartment. That seemed enough to activate my plan. I volunteered that, as her legal guardian, I would take full responsibility for her well-being and that I would arrive at Glengrove the next morning. By that time I wanted my mother to have had her hair and nails done, as she did every week. And I wanted her in a fresh dress, one that she liked. I would stay with her for two days, after which I asked for a meeting of senior staff to determine whether she was competent enough to remain a resident in her apartment. I requested that the meeting be held in the boardroom of the apartments, not in the "sick building."

Susan was aware of and agreed to this plan. She arranged for the beauty parlor appointment and even helped my mother pick out a dress. "Residents," said Susan, "need advocates."

I arrived the next day, drove to Glengrove, and took the elevator to my mother's apartment. I was told she was in the beauty salon, a few doors down the hall. I saw her having her hair and nails done. When I walked in, she must have sensed I was there, because she turned around, and the biggest and brightest smile appeared on her face. I felt great. My mother was home.

I asked our friend Lynn, my brother's widow, Barbara, and Barbara's mother to bring a Chinese dinner to the apartment. I was eager for my mother to feel comfortable, to be around friends. She seemed happy but also apprehensive: would she be sent back to the "sick building"? I assured her that she was home to stay. This proved to be a promise I could not keep.

That day and the next went smoothly. The afternoon of the second day brought the meeting. I told my mother that its purpose was only to confirm that she was quite able to function in her apartment. No one, I said, would force her out. Susan, Dr.

Linda, the head nurse, and a social worker from the skilled nursing unit—along with my mother and I—were seated around a table in the conference room. Dr. Linda said a businesslike hello to my mother and me—and then nothing else. I saw my mother, a proud and independent person, do something I had never seen before: she bowed her head, as if in submission, and said nothing. She replied to gentle questions from Susan and me with a nod. Dr. Linda only stared at her.

The meeting lasted only a few minutes. At the end of it, I asked my mother whether she felt comfortable in her apartment. She quietly said yes, and the meeting adjourned. The staff went to Susan's office. About ten minutes later, Susan telephoned my mother's apartment: "Your mother stays in her apartment."

That wasn't quite the end of the matter. After the staff had left, I met privately with Susan. I wanted to replace Dr. Linda, but I wanted to do so in a way that would not appear critical of her. I discussed this with my mother, who, with a bit of a smile, agreed. After all, Dr. Linda was an ongoing presence at Glengrove. At some point my mother might have to interact with her. I wanted no animosity.

I thought that the best approach was for me to take the responsibility for changing my mother's doctor. I had the authority to do this under a signed power of attorney. In a telephone call to Dr. Linda, I exercised that power. I told her that as my mother's legal representative, I saw a need for ongoing communication with her doctor, and apparently her practice simply did not allow for this. I thanked her for her services. Dr. Linda replied that she was sorry to lose my mother as a patient.

Dr. Linda was not content with my decision. Within minutes of my conversation with her, she went to my mother's apartment and asked, "Were you unhappy with my services?" My mother answered, "It was my son's decision to fire you, not mine."

I did not "fire" Dr. Linda until, with the help of Susan, I had obtained the services of another physician. His name was Dr. Stewart, and he himself was a senior whose practice was limited to the elderly—primarily those residing in the apartments and the nursing home of Glengrove. For decades, many of the patients had been residents at the Orthodox home. In a telephone conversation he asked me about my mother: What was her personality? What was her general health?

I was frank with him. My mother's wish—and mine—was for an absolute minimum of medical intervention, including the use of drugs. We wanted him because Glengrove required a physician, and we needed medical help in case of emergencies, especially a physician to visit her at the hospital should that become necessary. He agreed: "I come to Glengrove and see residents there. They don't have to come to my office. We'll see how your mother responds to me. I've been a physician to older people, and by and large, we seem to get along." Then he checked her chart and ordered that the medications she had been receiving continue.

I told my mother that I had employed Dr. Stewart conditionally. She had to be satisfied with him. But she had to understand that we needed an attending physician for her and that the choice of doctors had narrowed. A few days later, Dr. Stewart saw my mother in her apartment. He had spoken first with Susan, and she had noted when he would come to visit. At that point my mother had become somewhat forgetful, but her impression of Dr. Stewart was that he was "okay, but not exceptional."

For the better part of a year, Dr. Stewart remained my mother's physician. He saw her a number of times at Glengrove "simply to check her out." The visits were not all by appointment. Often, as he moved between patients, he passed the deli where my mother was seated at what became known as her table.

One day, to save time between patients, Dr. Stewart pulled up a chair next to my mother in the deli. He took out his stethoscope and was about to measure my mother's heartbeat. What he got was measured anger. "You are not going to examine me here," my mother said. "I have my privacy. I am not a child." She brushed the stethoscope away.

Embarrassed, Dr. Stewart left. He went to Susan's office and told her that my mother should find another doctor. The next day, however, he again visited Glengrove, knocked on my mother's apartment door, and said, "You were right. I'm sorry. From now on I'll examine you only in your apartment." My mother accepted his apology and a new, more personal doctor-patient relationship developed.

OF FALLS, THE HOSPITAL, AND THE "SICK BUILDING"

My mother suffered another fall and hospitalization several weeks later. On a Saturday evening, she fell in the corridor between the apartments and the deli. She was bruised but fully conscious. She wanted to try to stand, but the nursing staff had her lie on the floor. They followed a policy common to many ALFs: Unless a resident can easily get up after a fall, 911 is to be called and the resident is to be sent to a hospital for evaluation and treatment.

Residents understand the dangers that await them from falls, and there is a prevalent fear of falling. Institutions can help residents to protect themselves by offering programs that will enhance their balance, and caregivers and residents can be sensitized to medications that induce dizziness.[9] Such measures were not available at Glengrove.

The fact that my mother was only bruised did not alter Glengrove's decision to send her to the hospital. Administrators followed this hospital-first policy without regard to a resident's wishes. Residents' fears and disorientation, far from being a priority, were actually exacerbated by the emergency procedures—being placed on a stretcher and taken to the hospital in an ambulance, waiting on a hospital gurney for several hours, and then being forcibly subjected to tests whose purposes were not described. I say this not to be critical of the emergency team or hospital medical staff, who function in an often frenzied and overworked environment, but to suggest that the staff at Glengrove could have made different choices if institutional policy had been less rigid and more resident centered.

Unfortunately, the staff at Glengrove believed that they had no choice. The institution's policy was firm. Its rationale probably was based on cost savings coupled with a desire to prevent lawsuits. In the face of this rigidity, I wondered why the institution didn't consider offering residents and their families the opportunity to sign statements outlining their wishes and absolving Glengrove from any lawsuits if it didn't seek aggressive treatment for residents. I think that many residents and their families would have signed directives that stipulated that residents wanted to receive basic care and comfort and to be sent to the hospital only for life-threatening conditions. Under such a policy, my mother could have spent the night in the skilled nursing unit. Her physician could have been informed. And the next day he could have examined my mother and issued such orders as he deemed necessary. This is a procedure used in a number of nursing homes and assisted living facilities in Ontario.

But this was not to be. A nurse from Glengrove telephoned me to report that my mother had been taken to the emergency room of the Samaritan Hospital, about five miles from Glengrove. She knew nothing more. The only information she offered was the telephone number of the hospital's main switchboard.

Try reaching a busy hospital emergency room on a weekend evening. There was call waiting, transfers to places and phones where there were no answers, and people answering who did not speak English as their first language. I was a thousand miles away, and relatives living close by were not available. Glengrove had no regular lines of communication with the hospital and no employee or volunteer who could visit my mother to reassure her.

My mother's situation was hardly unique. It was all too common. A study of ALFs reported that 24 percent of residents sampled were taken to hospital emergency rooms within a twelve-month period, and 32 percent of those who received emergency-room service had overnight hospital stays. ALF residents' use of hospital emergency rooms, and the number of their overnight stays, were greater than that for the elderly population as whole (18 percent and 26 percent).

A significant number of the emergency-room visits were the result of falls. According to the same study 37 percent of the ALF residents suffered falls within the preceding year. More detailed statistics come from Canada, where more than 54 percent of the 197,002 hospital injury admissions in 1999–2000 were caused by falls. Well over half were seniors. In Toronto, paramedics responded to 22,000 emergency calls in 2001 for people who fell.[10]

In the United States, ALFs may be quick to shuttle residents to emergency rooms—even when their problems aren't genuine emergencies—because they aren't charged for ambulance or emergency-room services. Medicare bears the brunt of these costs. ALFs could spare taxpayers this expense by having RNs or nurse practitioners on staff. Experienced nurses could evaluate patients to see whether hospital visits are warranted. But this, of course, would add to the labor costs of ALFs.

Had a nurse practitioner been available, my mother could have been spared her second ER encounter, one that was particularly painful for both of us. Hours passed, for example, before I heard any news of her condition. I needed answers. I decided to fake a medical degree. At that point, as I was trying to reach a doctor or nurse to find out about my mother, I frankly didn't give a damn. I was connected, once again to the emergency room. In an officious voice I said, "This is Dr. Baum. Connect me with the physician attending to my mother—now."

Within seconds, I was connected with a busy and probably harassed emergency-room physician. "Not to worry," he said.

My mother had just bruised her leg and suffered a mild strain. They were going to keep her overnight just to make sure she could walk. She would be transferred to a ward. The next morning, a physical therapist would look in and probably have her returned to Glengrove.

I asked, "Would you mind having a nurse bring a cell phone to my mother so that I could say hello?" He answered: "Of course not, doctor. I don't mind at all." My impersonation had worked, and I succeeded in talking briefly with my mother. But what a way to establish communication with a defenseless and frightened elderly mother!

I thought that my mother's hospital adventure was almost at an end. There remained her return to Glengrove and the skilled-nursing unit, but we would deal with that later. I was wrong. An internist, obviously bent on procedure, was loose in my mother's ward. For reasons never explained, he ordered a colonoscopy—an invasive, traumatizing procedure for her. No one asked her permission. And no one asked my permission, though my medical power of attorney, I was later told, had been faxed to the hospital as part of my mother's medical record. No one bothered to ascertain whether she would give her consent or whether she had a proxy who would make decisions for her.

Following the colonoscopy, the internist gave my mother a prescription to treat what he termed a "possible" ulcer and an appointment to see him the following week. It was an appointment that I canceled, and I refused to order the prescription. My mother had never complained of stomach or digestive problems.

My mother was lucky. The colonoscopy did not do her any physical harm, though such a procedure has its risks. (This says nothing about the emotional trauma resulting from a colonoscopy.) Despite my medical power of attorney, I couldn't protect her.

In fact, even doctors seem unable to protect their families—or themselves—against the dangers of a hospital stay. In a 2002 survey of eight hundred U.S. doctors and twelve hundred other adults conducted by the Harvard School of Public Health and the Henry J. Kaiser Family Foundation, a total of 35 percent of the doctors said that either they or their family members had experienced serious medical errors in the course of hospital treatment. The errors had serious health consequences such as death, long-term disability, or severe pain. Three in ten of the doctors had seen hospital errors that caused serious harm to patients outside the doctors' own families within the year of the survey.[11]

My mother, shaken by her hospital experience, was returned to Glengrove. She knew that she could not return to her apartment until she passed through the skilled nursing unit—and that might take a few days. Dr. Stewart was there on the day of her return. His examination proved what he had suspected. Part of the reason for my mother's fall was dizziness. This was attributable to congestive heart failure which, according to him, was not an uncommon condition among the elderly.

To avoid falls, he insisted that my mother use a walker and that she use a portable oxygen tank. Her response was outright rejection: "A walker and oxygen are for old people. . . . I'm not going to use the walker or take the oxygen." Dr. Stewart tried persuasion to no avail. Reluctantly, he told my mother that she either had to do what he asked or she would not be able to return to her apartment. She would have to be admitted to the nursing home.

I had a talk with Susan and Dr. Stewart. He seemed genuinely concerned about my mother's health. He hinted at, but did not explain in any detail, the nature of congestive heart failure. I went to the Internet and learned that my mother's heart was not pumping effectively, which meant that her blood was not flowing as well as it should have. The life expectancy for people her age is somewhat in excess of three years from the time of diagnosis. Aside from heart replacement (out of the question for a person my mother's age), there is no cure—only noninvasive procedures to help her feel comfortable. The walker would help to stabilize her, and the oxygen would prevent dizziness.

Dr. Stewart had another concern: If my mother didn't follow his instructions and suffered another fall, he believed there was a danger of a malpractice action. He did not want to risk that possibility.

Susan and I worked out a compromise to get my mother out of the skilled nursing unit and back to her apartment. I sent Dr. Stewart an e-mail verifying that I held power of attorney in matters relating to my mother's health. (He was aware of this.) In the exercise of that power, I stated that I would hold him harmless for any injury that might result from my mother's failure to use a walker or the oxygen as he prescribed. Susan paved the way with Dr. Stewart, who, as I mentioned, was a person she had known and liked as a physician with the old Orthodox home.

I told my mother why the walker and oxygen were required. I explained that in her apartment she might decide not to use them. There was no one there to force her to do otherwise. Outside her apartment, however, at least for a few months, I asked that she follow Dr. Stewart's orders. At the end of that time, if she felt that either or both were not of real value to her, we would have a further talk with the doctor.

Dr. Stewart agreed to the conditions, and my mother was allowed to go back to her apartment. On a visit several weeks later, I spoke with Sylvia, the head volunteer at Glengrove. She told me that my mother seemed to be doing well, but she wasn't using her walker or her oxygen. "One day," Sylvia said, "I asked her why she wasn't using the walker and the oxygen. She answered, with a chuckle, 'I guess I forgot.'"

If Dr. Stewart saw my mother minus the walker and the oxygen apparatus, he said nothing to me, or to Susan. Weeks went by. It was really quite wonderful to have an absence of any crisis. Then came a call from Dr. Stewart. "Your mother is okay," he said. "The purpose of the call is to tell you that I am leaving my practice in a month. My malpractice insurance rates have gone up to $30,000 year. It just isn't worth it to me to stay. I really don't have any doctor to recommend." I thanked him and told him that I would miss him, as would my mother, in her own way.

The search was on to find another attending physician. Dr. Brian, as he preferred to be called, came to fill the position of Dr. Linda. He was young, new to the practice of medicine, and had an office close to Glengrove. Glengrove's administration referred residents to him, and, gratifyingly, he visited residents in their apartments.

As it turned out, Dr. Brian was to be the last of my mother's physicians. He was professional, but understandably he was busy building his practice. This meant that he had little time or inclination to probe my mother's condition or her needs or to readily accept my phone calls. What was more troubling was that the help that Susan so often gave my mother diminished. Susan had her own problems. Both her parents, quite elderly and in fragile health, had been admitted to Glengrove. Their condition rapidly deteriorated, and within a few months Susan, in addition to her regular job, was sitting a death vigil.

The following year, my mother had another fall, and this proved to be the beginning of her end.

6 The End of My Mother's Life

ANOTHER FALL AND A TRIP TO THE HOSPITAL

It is now three years since my mother died. She had lived at the ALF for over six years. Only two months elapsed between her final admission to the skilled nursing unit of the nursing home and her death. Although her decline was relatively swift, it has left an imprint with which I am still trying to cope.

As I said in the introduction, since my mother's passing, I have shared my experiences with others whose parents have died in assisted living facilities, and I have come to understand that my mother's experience was neither unique nor just a matter of bad luck. Rather, it was the logical outcome of a way of death that seemed to be almost built into the ALF experience.

Our final journey began on a January night when Sarah, an LPN, called from Glengrove's skilled nursing unit. My mother had been there for three days following another fall and visit to the hospital. For some unknown reason, she had pulled an emergency cord. Responding, Sarah found her on the floor. She had fallen again.

I knew that policy at Glengrove required that an ambulance be called to take my mother to the ER if she was unable to stand and walk on her own. I knew, also, that this would result in a longer stay in the "sick building" upon her return. "Isn't it possible," I asked, "for my mother to be placed on her bed or kept in the skilled nursing unit until her doctor can see her tomorrow?"

"Sorry," Sarah answered. "Your mother said the same thing to me, but she seemed to be in a state of some shock, and her breathing was erratic. We called 911, and an ambulance has taken her to the Samaritan Hospital." In other words, things had been set in motion, and there was nothing that either my mother or I could do about it.

Contacting the hospital emergency room and reaching a knowledgeable nurse and the attending doctor was no easier than it had been after my mother's earlier falls. To reach the attending doctor I again had to identify myself as "Dr. Baum." "Not to worry," the doctor said. "Your mother is bruised, but it's nothing serious. However, we did find her disoriented and confused. We'll keep her for a few days, just to check her out, and then we'll send her back to Glengrove."

This wasn't what I wanted, and it wasn't what my mother wanted. "I want to go back to my apartment," she told me over the phone. "I don't want to be here. I don't know what happened. I don't know why I fell."

"Mother," I said, "we all want to see you back in your apartment. Just give the hospital a day or two to check you out and make sure you're okay. Then you'll go to the skilled nursing unit at Glengrove." (I never liked referring to it as the "sick building" in my mother's presence.) I added, "They too will want to check you out. Let's hope it will be only an overnight stay once you're returned to Glengrove."

My mother sighed audibly. She seemed to doubt that she would ever be returning to her apartment. And she was right. The hospital stay was the start on what became a fast slide to death.

I did not then question the medical conclusions concerning my mother. Rather, what I found—and still find—so frustrating and anger provoking was the way Glengrove and my mother's new doctor, Dr. Brian, interacted with her and with me. They denied my mother's right to control the final stage in her life, her right to die as she wanted.

What she wanted seemed to be such a small thing, something that could, with my help, both financial and emotional, so easily have been arranged: "Let me go back to my apartment."

But my mother's last wish probably represented a legal liability to Glengrove. If there were a fall that could or should have been reasonably foreseen by the facility and injury resulted, there might be a lawsuit. If she were unable to take reasonable safety precautions on returning to her apartment and started a fire, again there might be institutional liability. For the ALF, a frail resident's return to her apartment seemed to represent risk without gain.

For my mother, however, going back to her apartment meant more than simply going back to the space she had inhabited. With its profusion of pictures of family and friends, along with her small collection of possessions, the apartment seemed to belong to her. It was a space she controlled. She could choose whom to invite in and whom to keep out.

More than this, the apartment gave her access to a community. Over her years at Glengrove, she had made new friends whose company she enjoyed. They helped her establish both a social life and a support system.

The staff at Glengrove endearingly called my mother a social butterfly. She thrived in the company of others. Even some of the strangers who provided her with services seemed to recognize this quality in her. Toward the end of her stay in the apartment, I remember a call from a representative of the oxygen supply company, which placed and resupplied oxygen tanks for residents. My mother had not been doing well. There seemed to have been increasing recurrence of forgetfulness and fatigue. (The use of oxygen was thought to aid memory.) The oxygen supply representative wanted to speak with her concerning the use of the equipment. My mother was in a common area with other residents. The representative said to me, "I just didn't want to interrupt your mother. She was having a really ani-

mated conversation with a number of other residents. I wanted
to wait until they were finished."

Continuing to be a part of this community meant living in her
apartment. The skilled nursing unit was not far away even for
residents my mother's age, only a ten- or fifteen-minute walk
from the ALF apartments; but for apartment residents it might
as well have been in another country.

In the spirit of the Eden Alternative philosophy of "neighborhood," Glengrove had made some effort to give the nursing
home, and its attached skilled nursing unit, an appearance of
warmth, a "small-town feel." The hallways bore street signs
such as "Holly Way," "Rose Garden," or "Tulip Drive." They
were wide and brightly lit, with many pieces of donated original
art (some quite fine) on the walls. There were small enclosed
areas, most of which were dominated by large television sets.
What the neighborhood lacked, however, was neighbors.

The ALF tried—to no avail—to encourage the healthier residents to visit their friends and acquaintances in the nursing
home. But most either refused or were reluctant to do so because this section of the ALF frightened them. My mother was
no exception; she too viewed the "sick building" as a symbol of
decline and death.

When my mother first came to Glengrove, her charitable im-
pulses prevailed, and on Friday evenings she volunteered to visit
the nursing home and light the Sabbath candles for its residents.
But she later confided to me that she found the experience unsettling. Residents with severe dementia shouted from their
rooms. The corridors smelled of urine. Eventually, she found it
so depressing that she didn't return. Former apartment residents—now effectively patients in the nursing home—were infrequently visited by friends. They spent their last days largely in
the company of other patients.

Bringing the patients to join the residents was possible only if
volunteers could be found to push their wheelchairs and stay

with them. Such volunteers were in short supply. Sundays and religious holidays were exceptions. They were special events usually involving concerts, performers, and the two rabbis. For the special events, volunteers in the form of students and adult members of Glengrove's volunteer corps were on hand to help. Generally, however, socializing between patients of the nursing home and residents of the apartments took place only if the patients had the capacity, on their own, to move about and to take themselves to the deli or the cultural center.

Except for Sundays, many of those in the nursing home were left on a daily basis to stay within the confines of their "neighborhoods." The nursing home had its own full-time activities director, who met with patients in small groups in the enclosed "neighborhood" areas. He seemed to be too busy to spend more than fifteen to twenty minutes with them. Sometimes he would simply be a kind of newscaster, giving that day's news highlights. Other times, he told jokes, which my mother, with a bit of a smile, rated as ranging from "bad" to "awful." (I thought some of the jokes were so bad as to border on being funny.)

The dining room in the apartment complex had been a social beehive, with mealtimes an important event. Mealtimes in the nursing home could not have been more different. The dining area consisted of a number of small, warm, well-appointed rooms. Most patients waited to be taken there, often by wheelchair. Others were served and assisted in eating in their rooms. In the dining room there was limited socializing.

When my mother stayed in the "sick building," both she and I noticed the difference between the patients' rooms and the apartments. Most of the furnishings in the nursing home were the institution's property. Patients were not permitted to bring their own furnishings other than, perhaps, a chair and pictures to hang. There was a door to each room, but it was a swinging door without a lock. Staff and other patients (and even their guests) could freely enter the rooms.

But neither shut doors nor interior decoration nor "neighborhood" activities could block the sounds and smells of individual decline. When my mother was in the nursing home, she heard both confused voices and angry shouts from behind closed doors and in the corridors. No amount of disinfectant or room spray could fully mask the smell of incontinence, even in this upscale nursing home which was far better than many.

For patients in the nursing home, LPNs and aides provided not only assistance but community. Indeed, there were LPNs and aides in abundance. However, they were so busy that I seldom saw them casually walking down the corridors. They were a scurrying group of workers with numerous patients. The aides were assigned many jobs that had to be completed before the end of their shifts. Medications were constantly being administered, following a strict schedule. They had to meet the physical needs of patients, ranging from bathing to dressing.

The staff of the nursing home were caring. With limited time, they did what they could to reach out to patients as individuals. Nonetheless, they were so harried that I seldom saw them chatting with patients. Given that the orientation of the facility was medical, socializing with their patients was something that staff could only do in their few moments of free time.

My mother understood that this latest visit to the hospital and her return to the "sick building" might permanently cut her off from her home and her friends. The social interactions that had so enriched her life would effectively end.

ASSESSMENT AND THERAPY: GOAL
AND REALITY

My mother stayed in hospital for four days on her third and last visit. She entered the emergency room on a Friday and was transferred to a ward early that evening.

On Saturday and Sunday the hospital had fewer staff. Like many other hospitals, during the weekend it seemed comparatively empty of both staff and patients. No staff were on hand to help my mother use her walker, though she was given some further blood tests, with negative results. Her frequent requests to use her walker alone were denied. Staff were concerned that she might fall.

This seemed to be part of a self-fulfilling prophecy con-structed by the nursing home and abetted by hospital staff. No one would let my mother walk, or help her to do so, because she might fall. During these three days, this ninety-six-year-old woman would lose additional muscle tone and become even more unsteady on her feet—and more likely to fall.

That Monday, late in the afternoon, she was released and taken by ambulance (the hospital's required method of trans-portation) to Glengrove's skilled nursing unit. On her return to the "sick building" I again tried to obtain a walker for her use. Again this was denied. The reason: the physical therapist would have to do an evaluation, and she would not be available for two days: her schedule was full. My mother would remain immobile.

On the first night in the skilled nursing unit, my mother tried to get out of bed to walk to the bathroom. Her legs were weak (as even mine would be if I hadn't been able to walk for four days), and she fell. The ALF immediately called me. Thankfully, the nurse at the other end said, "We're not sending her to the hospital. She didn't hurt herself. But we wanted you to know and to understand why we can't allow her to use a walker." I answered, "If she isn't encouraged to walk and given assistance, then the chances are she won't be able to walk." "Well," the nurse replied, "I'll be sure to let the physical therapist know how you feel."

Who was the physical therapist? I wondered. What was her role in caring for my mother, and what care program were they following? Was it designed to lead to her maximum well-being and facilitate a return to her apartment?

I wrongly assumed that, following assessment, the raison d'être of the skilled nursing unit was to design and implement a patient-care plan. At no point, either in this admission or in my mother's past stays in the unit, was I told of the procedures for assessment, a patient-care plan, or implementation of that plan —all required by law.

I was told only that the nursing staff, led by the physical therapist who would perhaps seek advice from her doctor, would both assist my mother and monitor her progress with a view toward getting her back to her apartment. All that the attending nurses told my mother was "We're doing the best we can. We can't let you use the walker because you might fall. Then it's back to the hospital—and that's not good, dear!"

For almost a week following my mother's admission to the skilled nursing unit, I tried to reach the physical therapist. She was not in her office. Voice messages indicated that she could be paged, but she never answered my frequent page requests. Only in the second week of my mother's stay did I learn that there was, in fact, no physical therapist on staff. The person who held that position had left the employ of Glengrove the week before my mother entered the skilled nursing unit.

This meant that no one from Glengrove could assess my mother's ability to move about. Dr. Brian did tell me, however, on several occasions that it was his firm opinion that she should not go back to her apartment. "She needs the care of the nursing home," he said. "She wouldn't be safe in her apartment." In his view, the combination of congestive heart failure and the "likelihood" of Alzheimer's disease (or increasing dementia) ruled out the possibility of her living independently. Dr. Brian made these points in very brief telephone conversations, all of which I initiated.

I strongly disagreed with this conclusion. In one of our conversations, I told Dr. Brian that I had devised a plan that would allow my mother to return to her apartment while at the same time recognizing her increasingly fragile condition.

My mother and I understood that she had congestive heart failure, that her balance was fragile, and that she had memory lapses. We knew that she needed twenty-four-hour help each day in her apartment. I found out how to get that help. The state had recently been allowed exemption under Medicaid to fashion programs for care of the frail elderly in their homes rather than in nursing homes.

The plan made sense. The cost of nursing-home care was, and still is, far higher than the cost of individual services such as those of an aide or housekeeper. Moreover, I would continue to pay the rental costs of the apartment.

I contacted the county welfare office and was warmly received. I quickly filled out and faxed the detailed forms. There was a staff review and interviews with my mother and me. All seemed to be on track for approval—as long as the nursing staff at Glengrove agreed.

Then came the obstacle: the welfare agency social workers wanted input from Dr. Brian. His reply was a prompt and terse no. My mother would not be safe in her own apartment. It did not matter that twenty-four-hour assistance with medical skills might be available. He would not budge from his view. In fact, however, his opinion was not the final ruling on the matter. This rested with Glengrove and that, in turn, meant the nursing staff and, more particularly, the physical therapist. They had the power to find a way for my mother to return to her apartment.

This was a time when Susan could have been helpful. She might have been able to give her own opinion, and as manager of the apartments at Glengrove her opinion might have counted. Unfortunately, Susan had taken leave from her job. Her mother was dying, and her father had recently passed away. In her words, she was in "no shape" to intervene.

Now, in the second week of my mother's stay in the skilled nursing unit, I needed more than ever to contact the physical therapist. One had just been hired. My many messages brought a response. He telephoned and promised an assessment and a care plan within a week.

My patience was at an end. My mother's strength was sapped. Though she still recognized family, friends, and staff, she had become more delusional, forgetful, and dejected. And she continued to ask to return to her apartment. I wanted action, and I wanted it soon.

I wanted the facility to do what the law required. When my mother entered the skilled nursing unit, I held power of attorney for her and signed a number of forms, not unlike those signed when she was admitted to the facility. The forms tended to focus on the financial aspects of my mother's stay in the nursing home, my responsibility for all billings, what would happen if bills were not paid, and Glengrove's lack of liability for the actions of its staff. The forms were one-sided, written by lawyers, and not subject to negotiation.

However, for this formal contract to be binding, there were general—and ambiguous—promises about Glengrove's obligations. Here the promise was "The nursing home shall provide the services required by law."

In fact, however, I later learned that a federal law bound the nursing home to a far higher and more specific standard of patient care than that of an assisted living facility. That law, the Nursing Home Reform Act, mandates good nursing-home practices. This means, among other things, interdisciplinary, individualized care in accordance with a *written plan of care for all patients*, with a view toward each person attaining and maintaining "the highest practicable mental, physical, and psychosocial well-being." These practices, the law states, are not one-time services. Rather, they are to be provided in a seamless fashion.[1]

Under the law, the care plan first requires good assessment as a condition of patient admission. Staff are to gather data so that they can formulate a meaningful care plan. Without that kind of assessment, the care plan would be fundamentally flawed. For my mother and all others brought to the skilled nursing unit, especially if they were seen as prospective nursing-home patients, a realistic review of the individual's abilities in walking, bathing, seeing, hearing, and eating—all known as "activities of daily living"—was required.

The task of determining walking skills at Glengrove's nursing home was assigned to the physical therapist, whose job it was to determine actual and potential use of a patient's limbs. But because Glengrove, at the time, didn't have a physical therapist on staff, this was a task that could not be performed until almost two weeks following my mother's admission. By the time the position was filled and the new physical therapist was familiarized with her duties, my mother had sat in a wheelchair for almost three weeks, during which time she was effectively denied the opportunity to rebuild muscle and balance.

Along with measurement of the individual's activities for daily living, the law requires, as a condition for shaping a care plan, the development of a *minimum data set*. This set consists of objective data for the nursing staff, the therapist, the patient's family, and the patient herself. The minimum data set includes information on the individual's medical and social history, cognitive skills, physical functioning, environmental needs, continence, mood and behavior patterns, oral and nutritional status, skin condition, and medication use.

The assessment is designed to help staff identify problem areas. For example, poor balance, as was the case with my mother, might have been influenced by sitting too much, weak muscles, medications, a urinary infection, or a combination of these.

When I learned about this planning process, it became clear that in order to gather the required data the nursing home would have to seek input from Susan, who had known my mother over a period of years and had interacted with her on a daily basis. But to the best of my knowledge, her input was not sought before she went on leave. Indeed, I had the impression that the minimum data set was never compiled.

All of this—the assessment and the minimum data set—are a prelude to a required *care-planning conference,* which by law is to take place *within seven days of patient assessment.* During the conference, staff, the patient, and her family are to talk about life in the nursing home. *Nursing-home life*, as a subject, includes meals, activities, therapies, personal schedule, medical and nursing care, and *emotional needs*. All staff who work with a patient are to be involved in this meeting. This includes the patient herself—even if she has dementia—and her family. The patient and her family have the right to participate in and comment on findings and plans for her well-being. This is a meeting about the patient.

The range of subjects discussed in such a conference is not dictated by staff. The patient and family may ask questions—and expect answers—relating to care and daily routine, food, activities, interests, staff, personal care, medications, and how well the patient gets around.

The care-planning conference is not a one-time event. It is to be held at least annually, with reviews every three months when a patient's condition changes. The product of the care-planning conference is supposed to be a written *plan of care*. This is a strategy for how the staff will help the patient. It is detailed, not a list of generalities. For example, the nursing assistant will help Mrs. X walk to each meal to build her strength. And since many nursing homes—including skilled nursing units—have multiple-room occupancy, the plans are to address nonmedical problems, such as the incompatibility of Mrs. Y with her roommate. The patient must feel comfortable with the plan.

The care plans are to be reviewed regularly to make sure they work.

We never had such a meeting. In fact, I remained unaware that the law required the facility to complete a care plan until I had run out of patience with Glengrove's inaction. This happened when I visited my mother two weeks after her admission to the nursing home and found her in a wheelchair tethered to a large oxygen tank, which had been ordered to help her breathe more easily because of her congestive heart failure. The size and weight of the wheelchair denied her any capacity for mobility. She couldn't move it.

"Why," I asked, "can't she be given portable oxygen containers so that at least she can move her chair around the corridors?"

She might take the breathing apparatus out, I was told.

"But she could do that even with the large tank."

"Well, we will look into it."

I tried to raise the issue with the nursing staff, the director of nursing, the manager of the nursing home, and even the chief executive officer of Glengrove. My calls either went unanswered or were answered with "We're doing our best. Your mother is receiving excellent nursing care."

Convinced that I was being stonewalled, I contacted some friends who were lawyers specializing in a growing branch of the law called elder care. They gave me the names and addresses of the regulatory agencies governing nursing homes and advised me to write to these agencies and to send copies of the letters to Glengrove. I quickly wrote a detailed letter, copied it to Glengrove's chief executive officer, the local long-term ombudsman, and the appropriate state regulatory agency. As objectively as I could, I set out the facts and asked for help.

The first response came from Glengrove's chief executive officer: a meeting was scheduled the next day with the physical therapist, the director of nursing, and Glengrove's social worker. I arranged for transportation and arrived on time for the meeting. My mother had not been invited.

The physical therapist arrived late. On his belt he carried a cell phone and a beeper. He began the meeting by telling us how little time he had. There was a crush of other appointments he had to keep. It was clear, in his view, that my mother would not be able to walk, even with the assistance of a walker. That being the situation, there seemed little possibility of her having the capacity to function independently in her apartment. Her future, he said, was as a "resident" in the nursing home.

I pause here to say a few words about the respective roles of the nursing staff, the physical therapist, and the patient and her family. The primary concerns of both the nursing staff and the physical therapist are the patient's physical well-being. I use the term *patient* because it describes the status of most individuals in nursing homes, as I see it. They are the objects of a medical environment not unlike a chronic care hospital facility. The term used by Glengrove for those in its nursing home was *resident*. In some skilled nursing care units the term is *client*, which connotes far greater individual control over the institution and the care provider than in reality exists.

To continue: at that point the physical therapist's cell phone rang. He said he was sorry, but he simply had to leave. He would be in his office in about an hour if I had any questions.

His appearance certainly left me with more questions than answers. Had he adequately assessed my mother? Had he assessed her at all? If she had so little functional capacity, was there no way that physical therapy could help her regain it? Some studies have shown, after all, that even the frail elderly can regain muscle tone and function, with proper rehabilitation. Why did he order none for my mother?

The physical therapist seemed so overwhelmed with work that I couldn't help wondering if his diagnosis was an easy way to dismiss an inconvenient patient and thus ease his caseload. Indeed, his offer to answer any of my questions at another time seemed pro forma. Given his demeanor, his willingness to interrupt our meeting to answer his cell phone, and his hasty exit, I found him an unlikely source of help.

After he left, I turned to the director of nursing and the social worker and asked what had been done or was planned to allow my mother to participate in the life of Glengrove. I told them how much my mother enjoyed her regular trips to the deli and how she valued the Sunday concerts, joining in daily bingo, and staying in contact with friends from the apartments.

"You have to understand," said the social worker, "we don't

have staff or volunteers to take your mother to all these events, or the deli. You are asking for the kind of individual attention we aren't equipped to give."

The staff concentrated on the negative. Neither the physical therapist nor the social worker seemed able or willing to develop with me a different outcome. The purpose of the meeting seemed to be to shut doors, not open them, and I began to feel powerless to help my mother.

It seemed, in fact, that we were all caught in a circle of powerlessness. The staff did not get to know my mother. It was not that they were uncaring; they simply lacked the time. My sense was that assessments and care plans—which to me represented an assurance that the nursing home was following federal policy with each and every patient, thereby justifying its claim for tax dollar reimbursement—were just so much paperwork.

Four months after my mother's death, I received a blind copy of a letter from the ombudsman, addressed to Glengrove's chief executive officer and copied to that institution's nursing-home manager, director of nursing, and social worker. It stated, in part:

Based on interviews with residents, family members and staff, our office recently verified that a number of residents and sponsors had not been invited to attend the care plan meeting. . . .

As you know, residents and their sponsors have the legal right to participate in the care plan process. But beyond the question of statutory requirements, we know that relationships with providers usually improve when health care consumers are educated to assist with the development and monitoring of the care plan.

Obviously, I am speaking here of something more than mere attendance at a care plan meeting. Best practice encourages facilities to write and communicate a plan which is understandable to all participants and which is carried out with the full knowledge and agreement of the resident or sponsor. Unfortunately, during the investigation of this complaint, it became apparent that some of your residents and family members were not adequately informed to exercise this right.

Included with the letter was a packet of material which the ombudsman said "we routinely share with consumers regarding the care process." He suggested that Glengrove should "feel free" to make that material available to families at the time of patient admission. It was that material on which I relied in sketching the legal basis for the care plan.

The meeting had lasted for about fifteen minutes. I went to my mother's room. (She was fortunate in having been given her own room.) I was jolted. There, on the bed, seeming even smaller than she already was, was my mother, whimpering in a kind of sleep, softly repeating, "Mama." I stroked her hair and her hand. Eventually she opened her eyes, smiled, and said, "Hello, son."

A THERAPIST BY ANOTHER NAME

Later, after my mother's passing, I asked myself why Glengrove placed so much reliance on the physical therapist to assess patients and shape their care plans. Of course, he had the skill to examine and make recommendations about a patient's muscle flexibility. As an expert, with proper examination, he could say, as he did in this case, that my mother no longer had the capacity to walk. He could say that without twenty-four-hour assistance she could not function in her apartment.

What he could not do was precisely what he did—veto the possibility of creating that twenty-four-hour assistance. He had no special expertise that allowed him to pass final judgment, directly or indirectly, on proposals that could have maximized my mother's strengths. After my mother's death, I learned that both he and Glengrove could have augmented my mother's functioning by utilizing the service of a recreation therapist.

Recreation therapists are neither physical therapists nor social directors. They are skilled professionals certified for one-on-one counseling and motivation. More often than not, they work in hospitals. Here is how Lincoln Hospital in Davenport, Washington, defines the role the recreation therapist plays in its long-term care facility, which is an alternative to traditional nursing homes:

> Recreation therapy provides services to patients and residents who are having problems that may be helped with one-on-one intervention from a certified therapeutic recreation specialist.
>
> The recreation therapist may work with individuals to help them regain abilities in a variety of areas such as communication, cognition or fine motor control of their hands. By using such methods as visualization, meditation and other techniques, recreational therapy can help individuals with pain, anxiety or coping problems.[2]

The recreation therapist is unconcerned that the patient has only a limited time to live. The challenge is to help the patient maximize life.

I recently spoke with Dorothy, who has been a recreation therapist in Toronto for more than twenty years. She told the story of Bertha, a middle-aged quadriplegic given only a few months to live.

To the nursing staff, Bertha seemed forever grumpy. She seldom smiled, despite the best efforts of the nurses. With her one finger that worked, she regularly took her electric wheelchair to a solitary area. A sister and a niece came to visit a few times each week. They talked and tried to cheer Bertha up, but she didn't respond.

Dorothy was assigned to Bertha. The nurses felt sorry for Dorothy, for they believed she would only meet rejection.

"What would you like to do today?" Dorothy asked Bertha, not in the tone of an adult talking to a child, but of one mature person talking with another.

"What do you mean?" Bertha answered in heavily slurred speech, seeming to say, "Look at me. What could I possibly do except die?"

"Well," said Dorothy, "I have a trivet stand which we can inlay with these individual mosaics. I have the glue. You press on the tube, point to where you want the piece. You can try and put it there yourself, or I'll put it on that place, and you press down." Dorothy gave a number of illustrations. Bertha watched, then said that she wanted to try—and she did. Later Bertha was able to move the piece, put the glue on, and press it into place.

Over the weeks before her death, three trivets were created. Along with smiles and conversation, they were given as gifts by Bertha to her sister, niece, and Dorothy. Adult contact combined with new motivation, starting on the first morning of Dorothy's work with Bertha, brought a new beginning.

For Dorothy, this was the meaning of her experience with Bertha: "I don't know whether my role helped to increase the number of days in Bertha's life. I do know that Bertha died a happier person than when I first met her."

MARGY: AN "UNOFFICIAL" AIDE

Because Glengrove didn't have anyone who could provide individual help to my mother, I had to find and pay for that kind of care myself. Since I had already contracted Margy, I decided to continue her services, even though my mother was no longer in her apartment. Margy wasn't a recreation therapist, and she had no professional training in working with older persons. But she had considerable experience in working as a companion to those residents of Glengrove who were becoming increasingly frail. For six hours a week (two hours a day, three days a week), she took my mother for snacks in the deli and to bingo, or she just sat and talked with her.

After I had found my mother whimpering quietly in her bed and comforted her, I turned around and saw Margy standing in the corridor. We smiled, and she asked if she could go in and talk to my mother. While I waited outside, she went in and closed the door.

About fifteen minutes later, Margy brought my mother out in her wheelchair. The tiny body with the whimpering voice was a thing of the past. It was as if Margy had waved a magic wand. My mother was dressed in a colorful blouse and pants. Her hair was brushed, and she was smiling brightly. The three of us talked as Margy pushed the wheelchair, to which the large oxygen tank was attached, down the corridor to the elevator and then on to the deli.

We got sandwiches and drinks. My mother had her usual—a half sandwich (salami on rye with mustard and onion) and a diet Coke. A few friends came to the table and spoke briefly with her. Nothing was said about a return to her apartment. For the most part, however, my mother just looked out on a familiar scene, pleased to be part of it.

In time, Margy had to leave. She brought my mother back to the skilled nursing unit. My mother and I than sat next to the nursing station. From one of the rooms came the cries of a woman: "Help me! Won't anyone help me?" The aides, bustling between patients, seemed to pay no heed.

I stopped one of the aides and asked if she could help the woman. She replied, "Oh, Norma always does that. She's calling for her dead husband. She doesn't really need any help. But I'll put her in her wheelchair and she can move along the corridors." That effort seemed directed more toward helping me feel comfortable than toward helping Norma.

After the aide left, Norma sped out of her room, propelling her wheelchair down the corridor and shouting, "Frank, where are you? I needed you and you didn't answer." She passed my mother and me and entered another room. "Frank," she said, "speak to me, you son of a bitch, or I'm going to throw something at you, damn it."

Maybe the aides weren't worried, but I certainly was. I followed Norma into the room and observed her screaming at a man lying in the bed. There was no way he could answer her. His name wasn't Frank. He wasn't Norma's dead husband—and even if he were, he couldn't respond because he was in a coma.

Unfortunately, Norma couldn't tell whether he was dead or

alive, and in her frustration she grabbed a heavy object and was about to heave it at the patient. I shouted for an aide, who came in and wheeled Norma into the corridor, close to my mother and me. She continued to shout and wheeled herself into another room. Once again, the aide came after her. As my mother and I watched, she leaned over and whispered, "Crazy."

Norma wasn't crazy, but she was in middle-stage dementia, and she later was moved to the Rementia unit, one floor up.

Watching this and my mother's reaction, I didn't know whether to laugh or cry. On one level, this woman, wheeling herself in and out of patients' rooms looking for her dead husband, was almost comical. Mostly, though, it was tremendously sad.

Not surprising, my mother said she was tired. An aide took her to her room and helped her to undress and put on a gown. I entered the room several minutes later, and there was the tiny form I had seen earlier, curled in a fetal position and quietly whimpering, "Mama."

Gazing at her, I felt sad. My tiny but strong mother was gone. No longer could she be obstinate and unyielding in matters central to her. Now she was controlled by a nursing staff that treated her as a dependent child.

HOSPICE

As I stood in the doorway of my mother's room, an aide said there was a telephone call for me in the social worker's office from Dr. Brian. He was professionally polite: "I'm sorry to tell you, but I really think you should call hospice. Your mother is dying. Hospice will be of help."

I was stunned. I had just taken my mother to the deli. She and I had talked about Norma. How could my mother have gone from being dressed, alert, and even bemused, to dying? When I asked about these sudden changes in my mother's appearance and demeanor, Dr. Brian replied: "Well, that's not unusual. I told you earlier that your mother is suffering from congestive heart failure and, in my opinion, Alzheimer's disease."

I was too shocked to protest. He again urged a call to hospice, and he agreed to continue as my mother's physician.

When I hung up, the social worker volunteered to have a hospice representative meet with me. Dr. Brian must have had a conversation with her, because she knew that hospice had been recommended. "They're always in the building," she said, "I will book an appointment for you." This felt like a forced decision.

I wasn't told if other hospice services were available. (They were. I was having difficulty focusing and making reasoned decisions.) This particular hospice proved to be a caring, informed service bent on doing what was promised: helping the dying person and her family.

I met with Mary Beth, a registered nurse who was the hospice representative. She had a handful of brochures, each of which she patiently reviewed. They described her organization, which emphasized continuous care and family contact. Initially, I was concerned that this hospice was a for-profit corporation doing business throughout the United States. It seemed to me that profit and hospice care were not compatible. But Glengrove was a nonprofit organization where, at many points, the bottom line seemed to overtake its charitable purposes.

She explained that my mother would have a kind of privacy. No incident or medical condition would result in her being taken to a hospital emergency room. Hospice promised twenty-four-hour care directed only toward her comfort. If I had questions of any sort relating to my mother, there were individuals whose names I was given. They functioned as a team, and I had direct lines of communication. No more would voice mail go unanswered for long periods. The team included a registered nurse as team leader, a social worker, an LPN, an aide, a chaplain, and a physician.

Mary Beth told me that I didn't have to involve the full team.

I chose not to include the chaplain, a Christian, in the false belief that he or she might attempt to proselytize. That was a mistake on my part. I didn't know then that chaplaincy, though initiated by Christian ministers, had directed their energies toward the comfort of the dying and their families usually without regard to religious belief. And the fact was that the workload of Rabbi Nathan at Glengrove was heavy and had left him with little time for patient visits.

I was impressed by Mary Beth's intelligence, experience, and apparent commitment to serve. I decided to use the services of her organization.

Mary Beth then spoke with Dr. Brian and briefly visited with my mother. She quickly reviewed my mother's medical file. To our mutual surprise, she found no Do Not Resuscitate order. My mother had been absolutely clear on this, even before she entered Glengrove. "I do not want to be artificially kept alive under any circumstances." Larry, my lawyer friend, had drafted a DNR order and explained it to my mother. She had willingly signed it.

The order, together with other papers, was given to Glengrove at the time my mother was accepted as a resident. At a later point, following her first hospital visit, Glengrove's staff told me that the order apparently had been "misplaced." In fact, it was lost. So my mother signed another order, this time using what Glengrove called an "official form." But that order also was lost.

If another fall or incident had occurred and my mother had been taken to a hospital emergency room, she would have been subject to the possibility of exactly the kind of aggressive, invasive therapy that she so wanted to avoid. The lesson: there is a need for ongoing review of what is included in the individual's medical file.

Mary Beth prepared yet another Do Not Resuscitate order, which I signed.

I also chose to retain Dr. Brian. There was much about his demeanor and behavior to which I objected, but he had been her physician for a number of months. On reflection, I should have chosen a doctor who worked with hospice on a regular basis. Then I would have gained a better understanding of the dying process. The absence of food or drink caused my mother no pain. Her body was simply—and painlessly—shutting down. The hospice team readily explained what I could not comprehend. (Yet there was a concern: How was I to know that a balance had been struck between medications that overly sedated and those which allowed for both awareness and comfort?)

After my mother came under the care of hospice, the staff assigned to care for her—an RN, a social worker, and a health care aide—arrived within a matter of a few hours. They talked with me, willingly taking the time to answer questions. I felt enormously relieved. I would no longer have to negotiate a bureaucratic obstacle course to get answers. These were skilled and caring people who were committed to be with my mother until her death, and to comfort me both during her dying and afterward.

THE ROOM: "A FAMILY ALBUM"

The cost of hospice, Mary Beth said, was covered by Medicare/Medicaid. In one final effort to get my mother back to her apartment to end her days, I asked Mary Beth whether hospice would be available for people living on their own in the apartments. "Yes," she answered, "but Glengrove has chosen not to have hospice for the apartments."

Glengrove was advertised as a place for independent living. A condition of tenancy was the resident's ability to care for herself. If she could not care for herself, then Glengrove, like many assisted living facilities, reserved the right to ask the resident to leave—a process called "de-admission." Glengrove, again like many other assisted living facilities, especially those with nursing homes attached, offered to find new quarters for people who could no longer live on their own.

By definition, those receiving hospice no longer are capable of independent living, as defined by the ALF tenancy agreement. To suggest otherwise, so the argument goes, would be to turn the assisted living facility into a nursing home—and, one might add, would subject the assisted living facility to a wide range of government regulation.

To allow frail elderly to die in their own apartments, or to take more positive steps to encourage residents of the nursing home to join in the activities in the apartment complex, might have hurt the image of Glengrove as an ALF, and thus compromised its ability to market itself to healthy seniors. Susan and other staff members were constantly giving tours to potential residents. Would these visitors be put off if they saw people like my mother being wheeled around the corridors or being assisted by an aide while eating in the dining room? Would my mother and I have been put off by that sight when we first visited Glengrove?

Perhaps if the standard image of an ALF was a mix of residents with different capacities, all living together—or at least occasionally socializing together—our expectations would have been different. But most ALFs don't seem to allow this to happen and may even discourage any hint that residents aren't active and healthy. Other "specialized" ALFs, however, are designed to function much like hospices.

Given Glengrove's position on the subject of hospice in the apartment complex, I had no choice but to end the tenancy agreement and empty my mother's apartment of her belongings. Barbara, my brother's widow, met me at Glengrove along with two senior members of the housekeeping staff. Most of my mother's things went to Barbara's son, of whom my mother was fond. The remainder, with two important exceptions, went to the volunteers of Glengrove for auction—apparently, a regular activity.

The two exceptions were the numerous framed photos of family and friends, and my mother's favorite doll, Anna (named after her mother). These were taken to my mother's room in the nursing home. We hung the photos on a wall where she would be sure to see them. She was almost enclosed in a photo album of those closest to her. Anna was placed within view.

I do not know whether my mother really saw the pictures or Anna. Her eyes seldom opened, and when they were open it was doubtful whether she could see anything. I was told, however, that hearing is the last sense to go. So, I described carefully to my mother what was in her room.

About three weeks from the time hospice came to care for her, my mother passed away. In accordance with Jewish tradition, the funeral was held shortly after. My son spoke warmly and eloquently. He mentioned strudel, my mother's best-known pastry. He likened her to her strudel, crusty on the outside and sweet on the inside.

A number of my mother's friends from Glengrove attended the funeral, many of them in wheelchairs or with walkers. Susan was there. I spoke of the choice my mother made throughout her days. Wherever possible, she chose life.

With my mother's passing, I thought my relationship with Glengrove was at an end. I was wrong.

SURPRISE AND RESPONSE

After all my mother's belongings had been moved or donated to Glengrove for auction, senior housekeeping staff checked the apartment to ensure that it was in good condition. Sharon, the head housekeeper, in the presence of Susan, had pronounced the apartment "spotless." This was hardly a surprise. Even though my mother was in the nursing home, her monthly rent had been paid and her apartment had been regularly cleaned.

It was a surprise, then, when I received two invoices from Glengrove. The first invoice was for two weeks' rent. This was to cover the cost of preparing the apartment for the new tenant. That cost related to the time necessary to paint the apartment, lay down new carpeting, and install a new refrigerator and stove.

I immediately called Susan about the charges. "Why," I asked, "should my mother have been charged for this? After all, in the normal course, when a tenant vacates her apartment and leaves it in good condition, similar to when it was first occupied, isn't that usually the end of her relationship with the landlord? Nothing in the lease suggested we would be charged for getting the apartment ready for a new tenant."

"That may be," Susan answered, "but I have to follow management policy. And that policy has been to charge for the time needed to prepare the apartment for the new tenant. In our view, it doesn't matter that nothing was said about this in the lease that you and your mother signed."

The second invoice was a charge for two months' rent, dating from the time *after* the apartment had been prepared for the new tenant. This meant that if Glengrove found a new tenant for the unit, it would receive *double* payment for that two-month period. (The cost of her stay in the nursing home was covered by Medicaid. It had nothing to do with the rent at Glengrove.)

Susan couldn't explain the invoice. "That's not my department," she said. So, I spoke with the person in charge of accounts receivable. Her answer was not satisfactory: This billing reflected the "policy" of Glengrove.

"But how," I asked, "could billing for two additional months beyond my mother's stay be justified?" The answer was "We just do what we are told. It may be that after a few months there will be some kind of adjustment."

Those charges amounted to more than seven thousand dollars. If, at Glengrove, like most other assisted living facilities, the resident population turns over every two and a half years, the facility would, "as a matter of policy," be collecting two and a half months' additional rent for each of its assisted living apartments in that period of time.

When I tried to find out whether this policy was legal, I discovered that state law generally allows assisted living facilities to determine their own costs. State laws seem to govern only health and safety standards. I considered taking the matter to a lawyer and then to court. But that would have simply involved more money and time. Further, it would have done nothing for those families caught in the same "policy" net.

I decided to take a somewhat different tack. The community had a long-term care ombudsman, funded largely by the United Appeal and other local groups. It would have been a stretch for that office to even consider the rent policy of Glengrove. But I thought that a carefully drafted letter to the ombudsman, copied to the "boss" at Glengrove, Emily Hahn, might have some effect.

In the letter I hinted that I might even go to the media. Glengrove valued its local reputation, and to continue its fundraising it needed ongoing goodwill on the part of local charities and government.

I told Susan about my plan. Upon hearing it, she urged me not to proceed. "For a few weeks," she said, "there will be considerable disturbance. Staff and residents likely will be upset. In the end, nothing will change except that life here might become more difficult. In the final result, that would not help the institution and, personally, I'm committed to the institution."

Susan's point was well taken. If my mother had been alive as a resident, a public letter of complaint might have proved hurtful to her. But she was gone. There was no one to assert the rights of the deceased and their survivors.

I decided to send the letter.

Within a week, I received a telephone call from Mrs. Hahn. "Why didn't you call me directly?" she asked. "You know, neither the ombudsman nor any state agency has authority over our charges. Still, I looked into the matter. There has been a mistake. You shouldn't have been charged anything."

There followed what seemed a long pause. Then Mrs. Hahn

said, "You know, the children of people who have lived at Glengrove as long as your mother often want to make a generous contribution. You may want to think about that."

I assured Mrs. Hahn that I would think about a contribution. In the meantime I asked for and eventually did receive a "corrected" invoice. I never sent a contribution.

7   Assisted Living Can Succeed

My mother saw Glengrove as her last home, a place in which to live fully and then die. She understood, of course, that a serious medical emergency might result in hospitalization and death. But her hope was that her apartment would remain her home.

She would not have chosen Glengrove as a temporary residence—as a bridge that had to be crossed between her home and a nursing home. Both she and I believed in what we took to be Glengrove's promise that she could age in place, with care and security, until the end of her days. Neither my mother nor I fathomed the potential conflict between Glengrove's requirement that a resident be capable of independent living and the resident's eventual need for help that only a nursing home could provide.

Well into the second year of her residence at Glengrove, it is fair to say, my mother viewed the "sick building" (the skilled nursing unit) and the nursing home as places for other people. Her social world was a healthy one, and she was constantly on the go.

Yet time brought another reality to her as it does to most of Glengrove's residents: a loss of their apartment homes. This actual loss of home, earlier just a fear, could result from mandatory placement in the skilled nursing unit following an initial fall and brief hospitalization.

In the skilled nursing unit, as in the adjacent nursing home, my mother's control over her environment, indeed her life, passed to the nursing staff. She no longer had the privacy of her apartment. In the interest of her health, the staff had unfettered access through a swinging door to her room. Her toilet facilities were located a few doors away. Her clothes and toiletries were back in her apartment and not easily available. At least initially, she had no telephone access to friends and family. She was in a controlled medical environment. This was not her home.

Here an important question arises: how might the promise that an ALF makes to a resident, namely, that she can age in place, genuinely serve the interests of the resident, the adult children, and the facility itself? In this chapter I offer suggestions drawn from my mother's experiences. I do not come to this subject as an expert, an academic, or a practitioner. I see these suggestions as pointing to what ALF administrators and residents, or residents' adult children, might do today to ensure that an ALF apartment will remain a resident's home until the end of her days.

A starting point is the reality that while nursing homes may be needed, they are not required in the sense of being mandated by law. Where they exist, they are subject to a complex interweaving of state regulations and federal overlay designed to protect and care for the home's residents. These regulations cover nearly every aspect of the home's interface with patients— the number of nurses, control of medications, and care of residents at all levels. The regulatory scheme resembles that of hospitals, and it is not dissimilar from chronic care wards. (A nursing home serves as an actual home to its residents for a year and a half on average.)[1]

The interface between nursing homes and ALFs comes when the ALF takes on the characteristics of a nursing home. This can happen. If ALF residents are allowed to age in place, it follows that a growing number of them will in time need help with dressing, toileting, walking, and eating. Some may become bedridden. The more individual help is needed, the more closely the ALF, for regulatory purposes, assumes the characteristics of a nursing home—and the closer the ALF comes to being classified as a nursing home, subject to the regulatory regime.

But consider that the elderly, even the bedridden, are not required to leave their existing homes for nursing homes. This applies as well to those who live in apartments. There is law to protect them, such as the federal Fair Housing Amendments Act (FHAA) of 1988. It is designed to overcome the historic prejudice against those with disabilities, and it prohibits discrimination in the rental of housing on the basis of disability. Its covers landlord screening of applicants and deals with questions relating to an applicant's health. Once the applicant becomes a tenant, a landlord may evict only if the tenant poses a "direct threat to the health or safety of other individuals." The burden of proving such a threat is on the landlord.

In 2003, in its first such case, the U.S. Department of Housing and Urban Development, acting on a complaint of disability discrimination under the FHAA, dealt with the complaint of Melva Platt, a seventy-five-year-old quadriplegic who had hired assistants to prepare meals and help her move between wheelchair and bed. The management of the facility threatened Ms. Platt with eviction. It argued that she was no longer able to live independently. The department ordered the community to allow Ms. Platt to remain in her apartment. She had the means and the help to live independently.

Carolyn Y. Peoples, the department's assistant secretary for fair housing and equal opportunity, said that a landlord must adjust leases to allow disabled tenants "to live a decent quality of life." That could include *allowing residents to bring in home health care*—even if a lease requires the ability to live independently.[2]

It is possible—though as a practical matter not likely—that the FHAA might be used to prevent forced eviction from ALFs. Remedial powers under the FHAA are broad. More important, perhaps, is this principle under the FHAA: Tenants with a disability should be allowed to remain in place so long as they are able to provide for personal security and not be a threat to the safety of the broader housing community. (I am not suggesting the use of FHAA powers to confront an ALF that provides daily services to residents.)

But what an ALF can and should do, right from the start of a tenancy, is specify in the contract a definition of independent living. This will require information and discussion between residents, their adult children, and ALF staff.

Conflict with state policy might result, however, if ALFs allow heavily dependent residents to remain in their apartments. Some states require ALFs to evict dependent residents and move them to a supposedly higher level of care in a nursing home. In these states, the "de-admission" policy of Glengrove would come into play.

In 2000 the regulatory agency of the state of Michigan ordered ten residents to leave an assisted living facility near Kalamazoo. The agency claimed that because of their level of dependence, the facility was in fact operating a nursing home. Representatives of the families brought suit in federal court to block the order. One of them, the husband of a resident suffering from Parkinson's disease, said, "If I choose to keep [my wife] in as pleasant an environment as I can and ensure she is properly taken care of, I should have the right to do that at my own expense." The husband paid $3,740 monthly for his wife's room and an additional $2,000 monthly for three private nurses who rotated throughout the entire day, every week. The state changed its policy. It allowed dependent residents to stay in an ALF so long as an agreed-upon level of care, approved by a physician and the ALF, was in place.[3]

I did not select Glengrove as a home for my mother after a careful reading of a contract or in-depth questioning of management or the staff. My mother and I made the decision for her to take up residency on the basis of reputation. And this was not a bad judgment. Until my mother encountered health problems, her stay at Glengrove was a positive experience.

But health problems did arise, and they were stressful for both of us. That stress was exacerbated by institutional issues centering on one single concern: my mother's uninterrupted life in her apartment. Glengrove, her doctor, and attending hospital emergency staff had other criteria to satisfy. They had a specific frame of reference for my mother, unrelated to her as a whole person. Once she met Glengrove's criteria as needing *skilled nursing care*, that care could only be provided in the skilled nursing unit. Once her doctor determined she could not function alone in her apartment, that was the end of the matter. In his view, her only available lodging was in the nursing home. Once the hospital emergency-room doctor received my mother for care, he administered an aggressive treatment that prolonged her stay, and he subjected her to tests that heightened her discomfort. There was no way for me to challenge their fragmented approach to my mother and move toward a more holistic one centered on her independent living and her comfort.

Realistically, I doubt that my mother or I could have clarified our expectations and assumptions concerning life at Glengrove. A careful reading of Glengrove's contract of residence would have given us slight indication of the facility's detailed "de-admission" and "independent living" policy.

(Very different conditions apply to those admitted to ALF facilities with Alzheimer units. Under state law these units have enhanced care levels and room separation to the extent necessary for the protection of the Alzheimer resident. The adult child and the resident are more fully informed of the conditions for the resident's tenancy. At Glengrove, the Alzheimer unit was made part of the nursing home probably because the required nursing staff was not otherwise available.)

Yet, what my mother experienced and what eventually led to her forced removal to the nursing home was part of the daily life of the institution. Exiting an apartment and entering the nursing home may have been painful and unpleasant for her, but in the institution's view it was all simply a matter of course.

On reflection, I believe that the institution concluded it was doing both my mother and me a real service by opening its nursing home to her. Because she had been a resident in the assisted living facility, she had priority status to enter the nursing home. In Glengrove's view, heightened care would be administered on a daily basis, for which my mother's heightened dependency was a small price to pay.

A resident's move from her apartment to the nursing home may come as a surprise to the resident and to her family. Sometimes the institution, too, is surprised, when its decisions provoke trauma and anger. What can be done to eliminate, as much as possible, this element of surprise? An answer, as I noted, is education, both before and after a residence contract is signed. The prospective resident, her family, and the institution must ask questions and get answers.

A starting point is to set a context for the questioning, which is not a courtroom procedure or a business negotiation like the purchase of a home. Rather, the aim of the questioning is to establish a basis for a *long-term living relationship*.

I wish I could say that I acted on the suggestions that follow. The fact is, as I said earlier, my mother and I chose Glengrove on the basis of hearsay reputation, visual inspections, and pleasant (but not searching) interviews—the way most people choose ALFs. The suggestions that follow are the result of hindsight. My hope is that others considering assisted living will benefit from them.

The ALF management comes to the discussion with the following questions: (1) What is the health of the applicant? Is she capable of living on her own, physically and emotionally? (2) What is her *attitude*? Is she upbeat or depressed? Will she add to or detract from a positive *community environment*? (3) Does the applicant and/or her guarantors have the ability to sustain her financially on a long-term basis? (4) Will her family be a source of psychological support to her? (5) Will her relatives turn into a problem for the institution? That is, will they be constant complainers, or will they cooperate with the institution?

What the applicant and her family must understand is that an

ALF under consideration need not be the only choice. There are other ALFs, and there are other assisted living possibilities. Indeed, I have made such a choice for myself, as I describe in the next chapter.

Without a felt need to move into a particular ALF, the applicant and her family will experience less stress. And they may also gain bargaining power: the ALF will see that this applicant is no sure customer.

One additional point about the discussion: questions ought to be asked of—and answered by—persons in authority in the ALF. For my mother and me, that person at Glengrove was Susan, the manager of the apartments. Her input was just fine, but she could speak with authority only about the apartments. She had no power over matters involving the nursing home. She could state her views, but the manager of the nursing home did not have to accept them.

What comes from discussion, ideally, is full understanding. For my mother and for me, the most important part of that understanding would have been a more precise meaning of the contract right to "live in place" or "live independently." Let's assume that Susan and the manager of the nursing home agreed that if my mother needed assistance to live in her apartment, she would be permitted to do so—but the nature of that assistance would have to be approved by the residence manager, and the costs incident to it would have to be borne by me as guarantor. Would this arrangement have been binding on Glengrove? The answer is no, if it was simply a verbal agreement that might be extremely difficult to later prove.

A written understanding interpreting a contractual right to *live in place* or *live independently* is needed. It should be signed by the ALF's chief executive officer, attached to the contract of tenancy, and made a part of the resident's file. If the apartment manager, the manager of the nursing home, or even the CEO leaves the facility (as they well might), a written, binding agreement would still exist. Such an understanding could be vital to the resident and her family at a later point when the right to die in place becomes important, as it did with my mother. (Of course, it is entirely possible that the CEO would not sign such an agreement. This should prompt the resident and her adult children to ask themselves, Is this the kind of ALF in which to live out the rest of one's life?)

There are other questions that should be raised—questions applicable to all assisted living facilities. It would be useful for consumers if ALFs were required to supply annual responses to these questions, which state agencies would then, in a timely way, place online for the public. If state regulatory agencies will not initiate such reporting, then the questions could be posed in interviews between the applicant, her family, and the ALF staff. The fact is, however, that the staff would not be required to know or speak as fully and truthfully as the ALF itself in a government-required response.

If, using a computer in the comfort of their home, the potential resident and her relatives could examine information about specific ALFs and the industry generally, this might allow for more informed reflection. Is an ALF worth considering as an option? What further questions should be explored in an interview with a particular ALF? On the basis of online responses, how capable is the ALF in meeting an applicant's needs, that is, her personalized care program?

The queries would impose no heavy workload on ALFs, and their responses would betray no trade secrets. The questions would include: the existing number of residential units and their description; and the number of employees, their skills (including certifications and training in understanding the nature of aging), job turnover, and shift placement (e.g., how many are on duty during the evening shift?). All have a bearing on the quality of life at an ALF.

Senior staff at ALFs have significant responsibilities regarding residents' lives. Information as to their duties, their skills, and seniority is necessary. Are there registered nurses on regular

duty? If so, what are their shifts? Do they have special certification in geriatric nursing? To what extent are the duties of a registered nurse performed by a licensed practical nurse? In this regard, identify who has responsibility for medications and
blood-pressure and weight readings. Also, does the ALF have
physical therapists and recreation therapists on regular duty?

Related to staff qualification and numbers is the matter of
how emergencies are handled. Who responds to residents'
alarms (pulling an emergency cord or pushing a "help" button)?
What is the staff's ability and willingness to administer CPR or
defibrillation? Under what circumstances will an ambulance be
ordered?

Who is responsible for keeping medical records? How does
the applicant know what is in her medical file? As I mentioned,
when my mother entered Glengrove I handed over, at my
mother's request, a Do Not Resuscitate order (DNR), yet that
order was misplaced or lost, not once but twice. Residents expect to end their days in the ALF. It is essential to know that
DNR orders are on file and available to the institution and hospitals to avoid unwanted aggressive end-of-life treatments.

How well the ALF functions depends, in part, on the quality
and stability of its management. Questions should be asked regarding the ownership of the ALF (for-profit or not-for-profit)
and the qualifications and lengths of service of its senior management.

And, of course, there is the matter of costs. What are the current and past rents (over five years), as well as service fees? Is
there consultation with residents in advance of any rent or service charge increases?

In the absence of government retrieval and posting of ALF responses, the primary means for information gathering is
through meetings and questions. The process can be arduous,
and the answers given have their limits. An accurate statement
of staff and senior management numbers and qualifications
does not bind management. For many reasons, the ALF may de-

cide to cut the staff, eliminate senior management positions, and even sell the facility's operations to another party. There was a credible rumor at Glengrove that its board of directors was actively considering a management contract with an outside organization as a cost-savings measure.

Similarly, the current rents and service charges may change at the sole discretion of ALF management. On occasion, especially when an ALF has unrented quarters, it may be possible to bargain for a cap on rent and service charges. But this is unlikely to last for more than a few years. When such a bargain is struck, it should be in writing, signed by the CEO and attached to the contract.

ALF management has considerable discretion to operate as it sees fit. Still, such power is not absolute. Most ALFs are subject to minimal state regulation that, among other things, sets a minimum number of staff on duty twenty-four hours each day. But that minimum number may bear scant relationship to the current staff total. The point is that, as a practical matter, residents and their families must keep a sharp eye on the maintenance of staff levels and quality of service. They must be prepared to voice their concerns if those levels fall or if costs to residents increase inordinately.

In my view, concerns about ALF operations should be expressed through residents' associations and liaison committees of adult children guarantors, as well as (if necessary) press releases—after giving proper warning to the facility. In the final analysis, it is not confrontation that is desired, but negotiation: talking with staff and senior management to reach a "yes-yes" solution for the residents and the ALF. At times, however, negotiation can come about only when there is a perceived cost for not doing so, namely, adverse publicity.

To secure a quality life, one that actually fosters independence, the resident and her involved family must be willing to assert themselves, to become advocates. Again, I emphasize that this role does not require ongoing conflict. Rather, it requires having a sense of what is important to individual dignity and enhancement of quality of life, finding the means to express oneself, and having the assurance that what is said will be fully and fairly considered.

Residents and their families taking the role of advocates can have a positive effect on an ALF. They can make suggestions for improvement and—especially in the case of high-end ALFs—they may provide added money to implement those suggestions. Consider the matter of residents' falls. At Glengrove, as at many other ALFs, a fall is treated as an emergency which, especially during the evening hours, is handled by a licensed practical nurse. At Glengrove, the nurse is under instructions, as a matter of policy, to call for an ambulance unless the resident is able to promptly get up and has no apparent bruising. The result: all too often the resident is subjected to unnecessary hospital emergency procedures—painful and disorienting for the resident, time consuming for the hospital, and costly to the government.

How different the result might be if a registered geriatric nurse were on duty 24/7 at the ALF with a different set of instructions. Suppose the ALF resident, at the time of her admission, had signed a clear statement requesting that any fall be treated solely in terms of maintaining her comfort until she was seen the next day by her physician. Or, putting the matter somewhat more strongly, suppose the resident inserted in her living will the following provision: "No person will direct this patient or client to an emergency room without the prior consent of the guardian, unless there is an immediate threat to life."[4] The geriatric nurse would only summon an ambulance if the fall, in her professional judgment, was life threatening. The cost of the geriatric nurse might be an expense that the residents and their families would undertake as an addition to their monthly fees. This added element of care would likely enhance the reputation—and the competitive position—of the ALF. This approach assumes institutional acceptance. Without that acceptance, even a geriatric nurse might well be conflicted in decision making. She has a loyalty to the institution as well as the resident.

There are other areas that call for resident and family input. The facility should explain staff positions in an orientation session for residents and their families. Such sessions generally are not held. There were none at Glengrove. My mother simply moved in and found her way among staff, residents, and the facility. There were the nurses (aides and LPNs), whose regular job seemed to be running tests for blood pressure and recording weights (at the request of residents' doctors) and responding to emergencies such as falls. These were people the residents and their families soon came to know.

Glengrove, like many ALFs, had a social worker. Susan had the qualifications (an MSW) and carried out many of the duties related to that position. She was highly skilled in helping residents deal with personal problems, including difficulties between residents and staff. Her job, however, was officially described as "manager" of the residence. She administered the operations of the building, supervised the health care aides, and submitted information for monthly billings to the accounting department. And for long periods she was the chief public marketer of the facility. The problem that residents and their families faced did not relate to Susan's competence or concern. The difficulty was simply getting her attention, even though her hours of work far exceeded those for which she was paid—and even though she rather freely gave her home phone number to residents and their families who wished to reach her.

Glengrove had another employee formally designated as the social worker, who had worked with the aged for less than three years. She was the social worker for both the ALF and the nursing home but was only minimally involved in the life of the facility. Most of her time seemed to be spent completing forms required by Glengrove. She was of some help to residents compelled to deal with government agencies for assistance in matters relating to prescription drug benefits and medical tests they could not afford. But her help did not usually extend beyond providing them and their families with the telephone numbers of the relevant agencies and contact persons.

From the viewpoint of residents and families, the ALF—and especially its social worker or the person filling that function—has the expertise to navigate the complex world of government (and hospital) bureaucracy. The reality is that this skill often does not benefit residents by helping them deal with agencies or cope with their personal problems. If Glengrove is any indication, a primary reason for the limited involvement of social workers may be a combination of heavy workloads and existing assignments not appropriate to their skills. Here again, residents and their families could contribute constructive input, even to the point of helping fund individuals on whom some administrative duties might be off-loaded.

Information gathering provides data to make that initial choice of an ALF, and it gives an indication of the openness of ALF staff and management to listen. It is a starting point for the resident and her family in their ongoing understanding and participation in life at the ALF. The reality is that for most residents of high-end ALFs, like my mother, the need for professional help is not initially apparent.

Let me illustrate. At the start of my mother's residency, she was introduced to the physical therapist. He, like so many other staff members at Glengrove, had held his position for only a short time—less than six months. By the end of her stay, there had been four physical therapists. My mother believed that his job was to help residents exercise. Twice a week he came to the residence and supervised mild exercise routines in which everyone who had a doctor's note could participate. However, nothing was said about more central aspects of his job. His office was in the skilled nursing unit attached to the nursing home. There, his task was to ensure that residents who were returned to the unit after a trip to the hospital were indeed physically able to return to their apartments. How he performed that job was not a topic raised in any initial interview between an ALF applicant, her family, and staff. Indeed, there was a clear break in the line of authority between Susan, the residence manager, and the skilled nursing unit.

The reality was that the difficulties of the physical therapist's position only became apparent to me after my mother was consigned to the skilled nursing unit. I then learned that only the physical therapist had authority to help my mother walk and to assess her motor skills. Only through persistent questioning did I learn that the position of physical therapist had been vacant for a period of weeks. Had there been open and ongoing communication between residents, their families, and senior ALF management, alternatives might have been found. Not the least of these possibilities would have been the families' hiring outside qualified physical therapists. Had that happened, perhaps my mother would not have been confined to a wheelchair and tethered to a large oxygen tank. At least she would have been able to nurture the hope of walking and having a degree of independence.

Only after my mother was in her final illness in the skilled nursing unit did I identify the kind of care that was singularly lacking. What my mother required was daily activation—stimuli to keep her mind alert and interested without regard to any inability to walk. This kind of contact was not part of the regular job of the physical therapist. Nor was it a role for the nursing staff, who were busy enough tending to the medical needs of patients.

It was a job for a recreation therapist—a person with motivational skills well known to hospitals, hospices, and even correctional facilities. These skills are applied—often with positive results—even to those facing imminent death or to those who are heavily incapacitated. The recreation therapist's view of her patient is that life continues until the end. My mother needed this kind of help. It was not forthcoming. Glengrove, like most

ALFs, had no recreation therapists. The person who came closest to having such skills at Glengrove was the activities director, and her focus was on group, not individual, activities. She also lacked the training of a certified recreation therapist.

Recreation therapists often are licensed and hold an undergraduate degree. They earn only about half as much per hour as physical therapists ($15.64 an hour in 2003, compared with the physical therapist at $28.22).[5]

In 2002 about 38 percent of recreation therapists were in hospitals and 26 percent were in nursing and personal care facilities. Others were in community mental health centers, adult day care programs, correctional facilities, residential facilities, community programs for people with disabilities, and substance abuse centers. About one out of three therapeutic recreation specialists was self-employed, generally contracting with long-term care facilities or community agencies to develop and oversee programs.

In the United States, there were only 27,000 recreation therapists in 2002, and projected growth from 2002 to 2012, according to the U.S. Bureau of Statistics, was estimated to be less than 9 percent. This data contrasts with that for physical therapists. In 2002 a total of 137,000 such persons were employed in the United States. Employment projections for 2002 to 2012 indicate faster than average growth of 21 to 35 percent, for an additional 62,000 such employees, a significant number of whom will be servicing nursing homes and chronic care facilities.[6]

For a resident to have a fulfilled life in an ALF, her family has to be involved. Life at an ALF is a long-term experience, and aging can progress slowly. The ALF, the family, and the resident should recognize that aging is a fluid process that differs for each resident.

In 2003 Jan Thayer, chair of the National Center for Assisted Living (NCAL) and president and CEO of fourteen assisted living facilities and retirement homes in three states, testified before a joint hearing of the U.S. Federal Trade Commission and the Department of Justice on assisted living and long-term care. There are about 2,300 members of the NAAL (proprietary and nonproprietary assisted living facilities). Thayer estimated that in the United States nationwide there are about thirty-six thousand assisted living facilities, serving a variety of needs. She stated:

> Currently, there is no standardized method for assessing quality in assisted living nor has adequate research been conducted to develop one. That is not to say that there is not a need for such research. There is. But identifying the correct assessment measures is not as simple as it may sound.
>
> The adoption of existing nursing home quality measures will not result in satisfied consumers of assisted living services. . . . A quality assessment tool for assisted living must take into account the active, independent nature of its residents as well as the more social rather than medical model of care, and must take into account the fact that residents' needs and expectations change not only as residents age but as new generations of residents enter facilities. . . . Adding to the complexity of assessing quality is the fact that seniors' expectations change rapidly as new generations of elderly with different values and behaviors enter the long term care marketplace. . . .
>
> A factor that must be kept in mind is that assisted living, like some other long term care options, is in the business of supporting and caring for people, not necessarily curing them. In many facets of our society from academia to government to the marketplace we tend to avoid issues of aging such as its effects and outcomes.[7]

A NEW BASIS FOR ASSESSING AND DELIVERING SOME ALF SERVICES

Perhaps it will be difficult, but *care planning* is a basis for setting standards and for measuring the effectiveness of an assisted living facility in meeting particular individuals' needs. Just as nursing homes must engage in a mandated process of care planning, so too ALFs in some states are now being required to assess residents, usually before and often no later than at the time of admission.[8]

The requirement, however, is of a "generalized" nature; regulators often leave it to ALFs to set their own assessment standards. California, for example, requires no standardized form, but it does require an assessment prior to moving in. That assessment is to include an evaluation of the resident as to fundamental capacity, mental condition, and social factors. The appraisal is to be updated annually or upon any significant change in the resident's condition.

Colorado also does not require a standardized assessment form. But state regulations require a "comprehensive" preadmission assessment relating to physical health, social needs and preferences, and capacity for self-care. (Importantly, Colorado, like Michigan, permits the ALF to keep bedridden residents, but subject to a requirement: a physician's order describing the services needed to meet that resident's health needs, including frequency of assessment, monitoring, and adequate staffing.)

Admittedly, the regulations in these states (as in most others) do not concern *individual service (or care) plans,* though one might ask what other purpose an assessment serves. One answer comes from the assisted living industry itself. A page of "Consumer Information" provided by the National Center for Assisted Living specifically describes what residents of assisted living facilities can expect:

> Each resident receives individualized services to help him/her function within the residence and within the community. Upon admission, a service plan is usually developed to coordinate the delivery of services to each resident. The agreement, which includes an assessment or evaluation of the resident's physical and psychosocial needs, is reviewed and updated regularly by the staff, and as the resident's condition indicates. The resident and family, or responsible party, are encouraged to play an active role in the development of the service plan.
>
> A resident care or wellness coordinator is usually designated to oversee the process of developing, implementing, and evaluating the progress of the service plan. A copy of the service plan is provided to the resident, family, or responsible party upon request.[9]

My mother was never assessed before she became a resident. No service or resident care plan, so far as my mother and I could determine, was ever developed—at least not one involving our participation. The only initial assessment came when she was placed in the skilled care unit following hospitalization and disorientation, which her attending physician suggested was characteristic of early Alzheimer's disease. The next and last assessment came during her final illness. It was given as a factor in her death.

So far as I can determine, there is nothing in state law that defines with any detail the nature of an assessment. And service plans, as such, certainly are not delineated. It would be good if state legislatures, by statute or regulation, codified what the assisted living industry seems to hold forth as its standard: individualized service plans developed in dialogue with the resident and her family and updated as conditions change.

Because the enactment of legislation can be slow, the care planning I will describe might more efficiently be done voluntarily. It would be a basis for real negotiations between a resident, her family, and the professional staff of the assisted living facility—as contrasted with the form contract of lease, which the applicant has only the choice of signing or not. (In all likelihood, that kind of contract would remain.)

I recognize that the suggestions I make are a kind of wish list, one that any ALF can refuse to discuss. But if some of the points in that list make sense and are put forward in discussions before a tenancy agreement is signed, it gives the consumer a further opportunity for informed choice. She will have a better idea of what to expect should she become a resident. The net effect of my proposals would be of benefit to all—the assisted living facility (management and staff) and the resident and her family.

The mechanism takes the form of an individual *care plan*. This is a concept derived from the patient care plan that the law requires of nursing homes, discussed in chapter 6. As noted, it is a concept apparently accepted by the assisted living industry. It could provide a means for the facility to remain sensitive to opportunities for growth and to anticipate or deal with individual risks. It is also a way for the family, the resident's guarantors, to express their concerns, to know they are not alone, and to obtain help.

Some words of caution: As a practical matter, for the care plan to work, institutional commitment and resources are required. Yet, it must be remembered that even under the best of circumstances the institution cannot turn back the reality of each individual's aging process.

The resident and her family need to become involved for the institution's programs to have a positive impact. A parent cannot simply be checked at the door and her bills paid on time, with occasional visits from adult children. The care plan is a means to focus on the resident's life and its enhancement.

The care plan, as proposed, depends on a professional team bent on working toward a single goal: supporting the resident. The team's mission should be to help bring the applicant into the facility as smoothly as possible. Under no circumstances would they be adversarial. The assessment team would become resources that residents would feel comfortable consulting throughout their stays in the assisted living facility, its skilled nursing unit, and its nursing home.

Let us now consider how the care plan could be used in assisted living facilities. Bear in mind that many institutions, like Glenngrove, operate both nursing homes and assisted living units out of the same physical plant. So there must be institutional awareness of what a care plan entails. In many ways, that proposed assessment mirrors the requirements of the care plan for nursing home patients. Some aspects of such an assessment plan follow.

Initial Resident Profile

To conduct its care planning, any facility would first make a careful individual assessment of a prospective resident. The cost of this may be an agreed-on expense of the resident or her guarantor, often an adult son or daughter. This evaluation would involve not only the manager of the ALF, the applicant, and her guarantor but also the applicant's physician (whose availability probably will be quite limited) and the ALF's dining room manager, social worker, activities director, institutional dietitian, chaplain, and senior nurse.

Why the dining room manager? No other employee of the ALF has such ongoing, intense daily interaction with residents. For more than two hours each day, seven days a week, the dining room manager deals with what most residents would rank close to the top of their concerns: meals. The dining room manager orchestrates the seating arrangements, order taking, and serving. She supervises the servers and responds to complaints and compliments. But more important, she has the opportunity to observe residents, to sense whether they are comfortable, and to judge whether they are interacting well with other residents and the staff. And she can spot problems. If a resident doesn't arrive for dinner, the dining room manager, who has keys to all units, can make a check. At Glengrove, the dining room manager saw her job as intimately tied to the well-being of each resident.

The applicant's doctor, if unable to attend the conference, could also make recommendations by phone or e-mail. A fee comparable to an office visit might be charged for that participation. With the applicant's permission, the physician would provide her medical history. The doctor thus becomes part of the assessment and also shares its end result: an understanding of the resident's goals and capacities and of ways to handle physical and emotional risks before any emergency occurs. The physician would not have a pro forma status, would not remain aloof from the patient and the ALF team's goals. (Some states, such as California, require physician reports covering specific subjects before the new resident moves in.)

The doctor's involvement in the applicant's assessment might make life at the facility less physician controlled. The doctor would provide relevant input, sharing it with the applicant perhaps for the first time. Later, when necessary, the doctor would receive—again with the patient's permission and participation—relevant information that would allow for informed involvement (such as a review of medications). The doctor would then be able to maintain an in-depth profile of the patient, one that would be updated at least annually throughout the resident's stay.

Of course, the assessment and its recommendations need not be followed by the resident after moving in. At the same time, however, there can be no denying that they constitute a plan of action to add quality to her life at the facility.

As noted, the assessment process would involve a nurse—ideally a senior or geriatric nurse. Tactful questioning during the assessment could yield information about incontinence, a subject of central concern to assisted living facilities and nursing homes. In ALFs such as Glengrove, we've seen, incontinence may lead to "de-admission," that is, forced removal of a resident from her apartment. It is also a subject many family doctors often do not discuss with their patients. At Glengrove, Susan handled the problem—often discovered by housekeeping aides—by chatting with the resident and introducing her to the use of pads.

Once there is awareness of the possibility of incontinence, the condition might be dealt with by a combination of exercise and medication (where appropriate), with or without the use of pads. The doctor would receive this new information and could monitor the patient through regular visits.

Ongoing Assessment: Resident

A resident care plan can have an impact on individual and institutional attitudes toward risk. Sometimes, as we have seen, institutional policy treats a resident like a child—it infantilizes her. Such a policy can surface in the institution's attitude about alcohol (not allowing wine at dinner) and sex (frowning on sexual or romantic relations). Of course, the institution may see itself as acting in good faith to "protect" residents.

For purposes of an individual assessment plan, I suggest neither eliminating nor approving such policies. Rather, I suggest that the resident and her family be informed about them before she takes up her tenancy.

Beyond institutional policies, there are individual matters of risk appropriate to an individual assessment. For example, suppose Mrs. Arthur, an applicant for residence at Glengrove, is a borderline diabetic, approaching type 2 diabetes. She simply loves chocolate, an unhealthy habit in view of her diabetic condition. Through careful questioning, the assessment team can become aware of such important facts about a prospective resident before her admission.

Here a doctor's input could be helpful. Mrs. Arthur's doctor, consulted by Glengrove with her permission, says: "For years, I have seen Mrs. Arthur as a patient, almost always for annual checkups. And for years, I have cautioned her that she must lose weight, and she must exercise. Her response had always been the same: 'If I want a piece of cake, I'm going to have it. I've worked hard all of my life. I'm old now. There aren't many years left. And if I want a piece of cake or anything else, I'm going to have it. . . . And I am not about to exercise!' So, as her doctor, I could only warn her. If Glengrove can do anything to help her live a healthier life, so much the better. But I wouldn't put any money on it."

I have picked persons with excess weight, inactivity, and type 2 diabetes for a reason: type 2 diabetes and its indicia have reached epidemic levels in the United States. About 20 percent of those over sixty-five have diabetes. Forty-one million persons in the United States are prediabetic. One in three persons who have diabetes is not aware of that fact. Diabetes, allowed to progress, is a leading cause of kidney failure, blindness, heart disease, and amputation.[10]

Yet, at relatively low cost, diabetes can either be prevented or controlled. The medical profession agrees that weight loss of ten to fifteen pounds and thirty minutes of somewhat vigorous walking daily will go a long way toward the control of type 2 diabetes.

Help of this nature will likely not come from doctors or hospitals. Five- to eight-minute meetings, or fifteen-minute annual checkups, will not turn around habits formed over many years. Hospitals have experimented with clinics and support groups. They have been successful, but the clinics have been closed. Why? The clinics don't make money for the hospitals. The patient can get meaningful support on an ongoing basis from a nutritionist at a cost of twenty dollars a visit. It is a visit that many insurance companies are hesitant to reimburse. On the other hand, there is insurance coverage for bariatric surgery (stomach shrinkage), a forty-minute procedure costing about fifty thousand dollars.[11]

Think about what a team at Glengrove consisting of a nutritionist, a social worker, and health care aides could do for Mrs. Arthur and others in her situation (and there are surely many others). They could set up a program challenging Mrs. Arthur to lose weight and to exercise by walking every day. The health care aides could see their training take a positive, goal-oriented slant as they help others enrich their lives.

Mrs. Arthur's family could be involved as well. Phone calls and visits could have an added purpose—to help Grandma get in shape. How marvelous it would be for Mrs. Arthur to have lost ten pounds and have a spring in her step. How good she would feel to see the smiles on the faces of her daughter and her grandchildren at the sight of her new vigor and, with it, new purpose.

Again, overweight and inactivity, precursors to type 2 diabetes, are used as only examples of what could be considered in a resident's meaningful care plan.

Ongoing Assessment: Family

A resident's family members ought to be brought under the umbrella of assessment. They have an intimate and lasting role in the life and well-being of the resident. For some, that role will take the legal form of being guarantors for the resident. They will be responsible for her financial obligations to the facility and a final resort should she be removed from the facility by "de-admission."

Yet, for all their responsibility to the resident, family caregivers all too often lack sufficient knowledge to be a more effective force. When my mother entered Glengrove, my knowledge of aging was limited. I learned on the job. Not the least of what I learned was the value of patience and understanding, mixed with a large dollop of humor.

Being part of a resident assessment process—and being in touch with skilled workers such as Susan, who cared for my mother—would obviously have been of help to me. Aside from fund raising, holiday celebrations, and the occasional lecture by Glengrove's physician, families were not part of a resident care program. Nor were other (but related) stresses of the family brought under a helping umbrella.

A clear plan of care would also look at attitudes toward hospitalization and end-of-life care. Let me make three specific observations. First, the death of Alice, who had become my mother's closest friend at Glengrove, caused my mother intense grief. Although she had endured the deaths of many close relatives and friends, in her later years none seemed to have had such an impact. I did not realize, until I studied some of the literature, that the death of those close to the elderly can strike extremely hard. I wish I had been better prepared to help my mother. I am not alone. There were other adult children whose parents (usually mothers) shared the same experience as my mother. Some of those at Glengrove—the social worker, Susan, the rabbi—might have been of more help to me so that I, in turn, might have been of more help to my mother. This assumes that they had time for such help.

Second, after my mother's first visit to a hospital emergency room, I became tethered to the telephone. Even on vacations, however short, I felt the need to be available. I had given Glengrove some alternate numbers of consenting family members who lived close to Glengrove, but somehow Glengrove's staff often misplaced those numbers.

More to the point, however, for those emergencies resulting in hospitalization, Glengrove could have smoothed the communications process. The facility was located close to a number of hospitals, and it had ongoing institutional contact with them. There could have been more than the simple message from Glengrove: "Your mother fell. An ambulance took her to the emergency room at Samaritan Hospital." The facility could have provided a name and number to call where patient information and hospital procedure would have been explained.

A member of my mother's team, perhaps a health care aide, could have been a regular visitor at the hospital and, later, at the skilled nursing unit, especially on the first day of her return from the hospital to Glengrove. The aide would have been a familiar and trusted face (in my absence) to ease the inevitable feelings of disorientation and, yes, fear. And the aide could have been a communications link with me.

Is it pie-in-the-sky thinking to suggest that a health care aide be a companion to a resident sent by ambulance to an emergency hospital room? I think not. Let me explain the rationale for a health-care-aide companion; how it is financially feasible; the positive impact it could have on residents, their families, and ALF staff; and a practical alternative.

Rationale. Unless a resident dies in her sleep, the reality is that she will be sent by ambulance to a hospital several times. Such was the case with my mother and most other residents of Glengrove whom I came to know. Each experience is frightening and disorienting. Not infrequently, close family members may not be available to reach the emergency room. How much less painful the hospital experience would be if a known health care aide would be in attendance for much of the resident's hospital stay.

Feasibility: To have a health care aide in attendance is a cost item. Yet it is a cost that the adult children or the residents in all likelihood would be willing to bear. It is a manageable cost. Compare it to the cost of so-called skilled nursing care, which at Glengrove in 2002 ran about two hundred dollars a day. This is what residents or their children had to pay when a resident was returned for "evaluation" following a hospital stay.

Obviously, the reality of hospital emergency visits and stays is something that management at the ALF should discuss frankly before any resident is admitted. The point is that, early on, a resident could opt into a health-care-aide-in-attendance program.

Impact: Frankly, the knowledge that she would be in touch with a friendly person, someone she knew, during each hospital visit would have been comforting to my mother—and to me. And for me, not the least of that comfort would have been the possibility to speak to someone on the telephone.

And think what it could do to professionalize the health care aides and integrate them into life at the ALF: They would have immediate and intense contact with a single resident. When a resident is in emotional need, they would see this and often be able to minister to that need. They likely would have the gratitude of both the resident and her family. A bond could develop between the resident and the health care aide. And since the resident or her family would be paying the cost, it could reasonably be expected that a portion of that income could be passed on to the health care aide as a premium over her regular salary. The position of health care aide would no longer be dead-ended and subject to rapid turnover.

Practical alternative. It may be too much of an institutional stretch to enlarge the suggested role for the health care aide. But there is an alternative, one that is widely used in one Canadian high-end ALF that I know of: privately paid companions.

These are persons, paid by residents or their families, certified by the institution to be companions to residents. They perform much, but not all, of the role proposed for health care aides. In fact, at this Canadian ALF (which incidentally does not advertise this function), the individual in charge of volunteer training estimated that 70 percent of all residents, including those in the ALF and the nursing home (about seven hundred residents or patients in all), have such companions. Some of the residents who are financially well-off have companions on a 24/7 basis. (The negative effect on those who cannot afford such companions certainly must be felt.)

My third observation about individual care plans also bears on finances. Admission of a resident to an ALF and a full life there hinges, of course, on careful financial planning. This is why any initial planning and the application process should consider how residents and families deal with financial issues.

In its application for resident admission, Glengrove, like most high-end ALFs, asks for information from the guarantor about ability to pay—including a general disclosure of financial worth. Even though it may be difficult to predict costs over the long term, a facility should be able to explain its procedures for any increase in rents or fees. So, in a broad sense, the institution would be aware when its costs begin to pinch an individual payer. At that point, the team social worker, along with an experienced senior administrative officer, could make themselves available to discuss ways the guarantor could continue to meet obligations to the facility and, at the same time, get on with life without risking serious financial consequences. This does not mean reduction of debt, but it may mean rescheduling payments. It may also mean sounding out community support organizations.

There are significant costs in addition to rent, the most important of which, at least until 2006, continued to be prescription drugs. In Alice's case, for example, those costs amounted to between five hundred and seven hundred dollars each month. For my mother, the cost was much less, but still substantial.

Confusion only increased for ALF residents and their families with the passage of the new federal prescription drug program in 2006. I am a reasonably intelligent person, and I have talked with reasonably intelligent physicians and pharmacists. Regardless of political leaning, they are hard pressed to know the best program choice for a qualified elderly person. I do not suggest that assisted living facilities are in a better position than experienced doctors and pharmacists to recommend plans. However, they are in a position to help residents make transitional arrangements until the administrative/bureaucratic tumult is sorted out. Many assisted living facilities and nursing homes have done this. Not to have acted might have resulted in physical harm to patients or ALF residents. And such harm might have presented serious issues of legal liability.

The point that I make here is that there are other programs, especially under the growing aegis of home care, for which assisted living residents would qualify. They could be of help and soften the financial impact on the guarantor or family. For example, when Susan determined that my mother needed private assistance, it would have been helpful if she had guided me to the support programs available in the area that—through federal waiver—would have paid all or a portion of the costs. This availability was not mentioned by either Susan or Glengrove's social worker, perhaps because Glengrove simply did not want government programs in its financial mix. Care planning, however, should include, not preclude, advice on this issue.

Assisted living is largely funded by rent and fees paid by the residents. (Ms. Thayer indicated, in her 2003 testimony before the U.S. Federal Trade Commission and the Justice Department, that about 90 percent of assisted living funding comes directly from the residents or their guarantors.) But it is doubtful that a facility could bar government support coming directly to a resident under a federal waiver program. I also question whether a facility could preclude its staff, given the nature of their jobs, from offering advice as to the contents of such programs designed to help residents *age in place*.

Assessment: Guide or Contract?

The individual assessments or care plans proposed here would—if facilities adopted them—function as guides, not contracts. They would be used as specific but open-ended suggestions for enhancing a resident's level of care. Of course, as I said, the facility or the resident simply could choose to ignore the plan once it was provided.

That is not a likely outcome, however. If the plan is carefully constructed, it will reflect the expectations of caregivers, the resident, and her family with regard to how the facility will help the resident and what the resident will do to help herself.

Because the parties in the assessments are not bargaining legal positions, they can speak and act openly without fear of their promises becoming fodder for a court battle. One does not take up residency in a facility for the purpose of initiating litigation. To repeat, the assessment would be used to set guidelines or goals to enhance a resident's stay. It would become something to strive for—a way to shape a team whose goal is improving life at the facility. Of course, this assumes a resident's continuing mental competence.

Nothing in the assessment or its construction should be seen as the formulation of legal obligations in the form of contract. The assessment is not a way to bargain risk. If Mrs. Arthur is told that eating sweets might trigger a diabetic reaction, then the facility, under the assessment, will not have absolved itself of liability if, for example, it serves a steady diet rich in sweets. Again, that is not the purpose of the assessments—though one can hope that Mrs. Arthur will be well aware of the danger of a diet rich in sweets and that the dining room manager, with her sense of self-discipline and the help of the dietitian, will act intelligently in her own self-interest.[12]

The assessment provides a minimal basis for an objective review by an enforcing agency. It can determine that a care plan is in place at the times required, that the requisite meetings were held, that the resident and her family participated in those meetings, and that the plan was distributed to them for their comment and verification.

In the Interest of Industry

What has been said of the individual assessment plan seems to square with the assisted living industry's view of itself and government regulation. Ms. Thayer, the spokesperson for the ALF industry quoted earlier, has this to say:

> The philosophy of assisted living involves providing the resident as much choice and flexibility as possible. *The resident of an ALF should be an integral part of developing his/her service plan, which outlines what services or assistance a resident will receive and when.* Because residents retain the right to refuse services that might be considered clinically appropriate, the end result may be that the residents' physical health declines more rapidly than if they had allowed certain care to occur. Still, the resident has made an informed and deliberate choice to refuse that particular care or service and that refusal is an important dignity issue for this resident. . . .
>
> A quality of life approach might say quality occurs when the facility honors the resident's wishes and personal lifestyle choice even though she increases the likelihood of physical injury. The answer is highly subjective and not easily discernible. At the end of the day, it is likely that either answer could be correct depending upon the resident's values, customs, socialization and the importance of this decision on the resident's perception of herself. This variability makes accurate measurement more difficult.
>
> Ultimately, it will likely be a combination of some process-oriented measures and some outcome measures that will be used to measure quality in assisted living. The obvious challenge is finding the right combination for assisted living and other long term care models.[13]

I wish my mother and I had engaged in better planning. I hope others do. The reality is that those who opt for assisted living for their parents will, in some way, be involved in their care and well-being over the long term. No matter how expensive the facility, and regardless of the promises made, parents cannot simply be left at the facility with the only commitment being one of paying bills. The first few years of their residence may pass smoothly, and they might be quite happy. As time passes, however, health problems will arise. Adult children will be called upon more frequently by their parents and the facility to respond to emergencies and crises.

My own experience has convinced me that planning is essential. I have made plans for my own future—and they do not include an ALF.

8   For Ourselves

MAKING CHOICES

Sometime during the second year of my mother's stay at Glengrove—at a time when she was especially happy with Alice and
other new friends and felt a real sense of family and culture in
the facility—she asked me, "So, son, what do you want for
yourself?" Knowing my mother, I took the question to be a kind
of invitation to join her at Glengrove. It was a good life for my
mother then, and she wanted the same for me, a single person
who had lived alone for many years. She framed the question
not to confront, but to prod.

I told her I loved her, but that my home was in Toronto.
Though I was by then a senior myself and had begun to collect
pension checks, I did not see my working days as having ended.
I thought that the perfect death would be a quick one—coming
while I was writing feverishly to meet a deadline on an important book. My friend Larry, a successful lawyer, said that he
wanted his life to end while he was in the midst of a challenging
case.

There are almost two decades between where I am now and
where my mother was when she entered Glengrove. I cannot
even begin to contemplate what my life will be like should I
reach the age of eighty-nine. Today, I can tell myself that I will
continue to be healthy and productive. My exercise regime has
been built over the years so that it has become habit. If I don't
exercise regularly, I don't feel good. So, too, although eating

good food and preparing it always gives me pleasure, my diet is sensible. My work is challenging, and it promises to remain so.

But I also know that we can seldom predict the future. I recall a warm summer day last year when I was rushing home from my favorite fish store, anxious to refrigerate that night's dinner and then head for the swimming pool. I ran across a street, stumbled, and fell. I couldn't get up. The fish and the other items in my two shopping bags scattered on the pavement. A young fellow helped me get to my feet. I considered either an ambulance or a taxi to a hospital emergency room, but then thought better of it.

The adrenaline was coursing through me. I had just finished researching and writing about elderly falls and emergency rooms. I had no desire to be another statistic, waiting hours on a gurney for attention. I had enough energy to gather my parcels and hobble home, where I bathed and bandaged my somewhat bloodied knees. It was my first fall as a senior, and it was, on reflection, somewhat scary. I found myself thereafter walking with far more caution and seldom running to beat a changing traffic light. I also became more keenly aware of my own vulnerability. And that made me think more deeply about how I would spend my own final years.

Those of us lucky enough to have the financial means can try to plan for some continuing control over our lives and our deaths. What I want for myself is to continue my life more or less as it is now—hopefully until the end of my days. I want what my mother at the end of her life was denied: some control over how to live, including—to the extent possible—some control over death.

MY VERTICAL NEIGHBORHOOD

Some may call it planning for a gracious exit. I prefer to think of it as being able to live in an environment that helps to generate enthusiasm, joy, and challenge. I have no desire to go either to a retirement community or an assisted living facility, where age is the dominant characteristic and waiting for death is all too often the dominant activity. I am privileged, even after handling my mother's expenses, to be able to finance for myself a different exit. I know I don't want to use my money to be warehoused with other seniors with whom I have little in common except age or income level. Recall that at some assisted living facilities/nursing homes, the annual 2005 rate ranged from $60,000 to $216,000. Against these figures, my mother had bargain rates. Still, in a short time, the savings of a lifetime can be spent—and on what?

Nor do I have a desire to think about how I can "game" the government by "gifting" my assets so that I can enter a nursing home cost-free as a ward of the state under the protection of Medicaid or its equivalent program in Canada—all with the help and expense of an eldercare lawyer. Money, at least enough to maintain my way of life, is necessary. It also helps to give me some control over my own life, and that can become more important especially at the end of life when one tends to become more fragile and vulnerable.[1]

Many seniors are indeed far wealthier than in decades past. But living on one's savings, whether in or out of an assisted living facility, will be no easy matter. Once we start to take from our savings in excess of about 4 percent annually, there is a real risk that those savings will be exhausted before our lives have ended. And expenses will tend to mount at the end of our lives.[2]

My solution is to use my savings to try to live my days out at home. It's what I know and where I feel comfortable. Although most seniors prefer to do the same, they often fear they won't be able to afford needed services to keep them safe and thus keep their children's worries at bay.

But there is a solution that may be affordable, both to the affluent and those less so. It's called a "naturally occurring retirement community," or NORC. Let me tell you about my home.

I live today, and hope to do so for the foreseeable future, in what I call my vertical neighborhood. It is a high-rise complex located in the middle of downtown Toronto, a city of over four million. I am where I think many seniors prefer to be: in the middle of a busy, bustling, relatively safe environment.

The rents in the building in which I live are, by Toronto standards, quite high. Yet my rent is less than half of what Glengrove charged my mother in the latter part of her stay. Moreover, at Glengrove and most other assisted living facilities, there are no limits to rent increases. In my building, fully enforced municipal regulation puts a cap on annual rent increases. (New York City also has rental ceilings.)

All staff members in my building—security, administration, maintenance, and domestics—are trained in CPR, first aid, and defibrillation. That training and certification, which is regularly renewed, happens before they are placed on the job. For example, a supervisor who recently retired after ten years' service was a registered nurse. Staff training exceeds that of health care workers at Glengrove and most other assisted living facilities. The workers in the building are numerous, especially the uniformed security staff. And they are on duty, with a minimum of eight security staff, 24/7, including holidays. Unlike health care aides, the staff here have been on the job for more than a few years, and they get to know the residents. (Recall that the staff turnover at an assisted living facility can be as high as 100 percent in a single year.)

There is direct apartment phone access to a security desk in the lobby, where a staff member always is on duty. Only the most senior security staff handle the desk. Each of them has between five to nine years' seniority. Next to the supervisor, the desk security personnel are the most highly paid. They are skilled at communicating with residents. The phone is answered within three rings. Some tenants subscribe to a med-alert service. If there is an emergency as the tenant describes it in her service contract, med-alert will call the security desk, assuming the tenant is unable to reach a phone. Security—usually two officers—will knock on the resident's door and enter if there is no response. The security staff is affordable because the commercial tenants share in the cost. Most condominiums and other rental buildings only have, at most, three security persons on duty at night.

A common type of emergency involves a fall. And here the contrast with Glengrove, and many assisted living facilities, is instructive. Security, once called and in the apartment, will speak with the tenant, if possible, and ask what she wants. Often the request is quite simple: "Help me get into my bed." Only when it appears clear that the resident has sustained real injury, rather than just bruising, will security call 911 and request an ambulance. The order of the day is to listen to the resident, a sharp contrast to Glengrove.

To be sure, there are serious emergencies that can threaten the safety of residents in the building. There have been apartment fires over the years. But there have been no injuries. There are sprinklers and smoke alarms in all apartments—checked regularly by staff—and a public address system. And there are alarm-testing drills. Further, the management office and security keep a list of tenants who have indicated that they might need assistance in an emergency. Those on the list are given priority response should an emergency arise.

What might appear as "little things" get done as well. Light bulbs will be changed on request. Dining room tables in a resident's apartment will be opened to accommodate dinner guests. Employees in the maintenance department change filters for air conditioners and heaters several times each year.

There is an administrative office off the lobby accessible to the residents. It is staffed by three seasoned management employees: Marcie, the manager; Judy, the rental manager; and David, the maintenance manager. Their seniority ranges from nine to fifteen years. They are highly competent and look after the tenants, their apartments, and the building. Within the corporate structure, there is ample room for movement. At corporate divisional meetings, the three often are asked whether they would like job transfers. After all, in these days of job mobility a lifetime job seems passé. Their answers uniformly are "No, we like our jobs. We would like to stay just where we are." At Glengrove, administrative staff turnover was frequent, except for Susan, manager of the apartments, and Anne, manager of the dining room.

My apartment is spacious. From it I see the city skyline and Lake Ontario, as well as sunsets. The neighbors are congenial, and the building, with over seven hundred units, is well serviced. I have been a tenant for almost thirty years, and there are probably more than a hundred other tenants who have been in the building as long. I have heard neighbors in their eighties and nineties say, "The only way I'm ever going to leave this building is when they carry me out."

We have watched ourselves and our neighbors grow older. There have been marriages and divorces. Children have been raised, and they in turn have had children. Indeed, grandchildren now fill the swimming pool on weekends and holidays. Many of us have moved from one career to another. Others have retired or chosen to work reduced hours. Many have taken on new careers as volunteers. One friend put it this way: "It's time we gave back something to the community."

Yet it would be a mistake to believe that all elderly people in the building where I live are fit and alert. There are illnesses, injuries from accidents (especially falls), and dementias, sometimes in the form of Alzheimer's disease. On occasion, as is true generally, the change can be sudden from apparent normalcy to serious illness. The difference between Glengrove and my building lies not in the kinds of dementia or Alzheimer's but in the proportion of the population so afflicted. At Glengrove, toward the end of my mother's stay, the majority of residents seemed to have at least moderate dementia. At the building where I live, the elderly make up only about a third of all residents, so neither dementia nor death are as visible.

Elderly residents live and die in my building. Sometimes, as with many forms of cancer, the dying comes slowly. The resident often is supported by live-in caregivers or hospice—welcomed in the building by management and staff. At such times the emphasis is not on dying but on living. Usually, families or close friends are on hand to provide support and supervision, as needed.

Notice I have used the word *we* for my fellow tenants. We in fact have a sense or spirit of community. A core of us have lived in the same building for many years and have shared the connections that flow as a result. During the great power blackout of 2003, which hit Toronto and much of the East Coast and Midwest of the United States and lasted for twenty-four to forty-eight hours, building staff and neighbors took care of the elderly. There was water, food, and companionship—even jokes and entertainment. Restaurants in the area served perishable food—by candlelight and at no charge. Auxiliary generators kept common areas cool. Later, when power returned, there were tenant parties.

Yet this is not a "seniors' residence." The owner, a major life insurance company, apparently prefers not to label it as such. The tenants are a mix in terms of age, gender, and ethnicity. There are students from our next-door neighbor the University of Toronto, as well as young families and singles. In many ways the tenants mirror Toronto. It is as if the United Nations had taken up residence.

The tenants talk and are, on the whole, friendly neighbors. Often the catalyst for conversation are the pet dogs that abound, ranging in size from Chihuahuas to Great Danes. Residents have come to know them by name. At Glengrove the only pet frequently seen was the rabbi's golden retriever. And at Glengrove the only generational mix came from visitors and volunteers.

The building is preeminently a people place. There are two gyms and a swimming pool in the residential tower (open from 6 a.m. to 11 p.m.). During the warm months—April through

September—there is a well-tended roof garden, with a ramp to allow wheelchair and walker access. Party rooms are also available at no charge, and guest suites accommodate overnight visitors at moderate rates. The elevators and entranceways are electronically controlled to give maximum time for people to pass. (They are wheelchair accessible.)

The building itself is part of a larger complex, also owned and operated by the insurance company. The residence opens onto a multilevel mall which houses restaurants, coffee shops, snack bars, a large bookstore, beauty salons, a movie complex with twelve screens, a supermarket, a post office, a bank (with special seating and service for seniors), a liquor store, and numerous specialty shops. Less than two blocks away are two world-class museums. There is underground wheelchair access to a good subway system, with the symphony hall, opera house, and theater district minutes away.

Marcie and Judy, who describe the building's residents as a community, use the words *eclectic* and *alive*. And they are right. Unlike Glengrove's claim to be a neighborhood, my vertical neighborhood has people who really care for and about one another. Marcie told me about someone who had been a resident at a nearby high-end assisted living facility: "She's in her eighties. It looked nice and secure. It was close to shops. But she said life there was boring. People seemed to sit all day in wheelchairs, and wait only for the next meal. She moved [to the building where I live] after hearing about it from friends. It's a building where the people and the environment are alive."

This community where I live is not planned from the top down. People with physical means and professional support have fashioned their own environment. The residents have a keen interest in this environment and the way it is maintained. They take initiatives, individually and collectively. A few years ago there was a rent increase beyond the annual amount allowed—as the law permits, for example, when a building requires major repairs. Residents discussed it among themselves and in a residents' association meeting. They appealed the action to a government rent control agency—with a measure of success. This could not have happened at Glengrove or at most other assisted living facilities.

Some people might respond that communities like this can work only in a vertical neighborhood, in a high-rise, and not in a horizontal urban environment with row houses or detached houses. And they might insist that a NORC would be entirely unworkable in a suburban community.

I'm not an expert in the field, but I do know that even in the suburbs, people want to remain in their homes if they can. One spouse—usually the husband—dies before the other, but the widow (or widower) stays on. This has been her home. What can come from this change in life for her and others is a NORC consisting of largely single-family homes.[3]

For example, the Boston neighborhood of Beacon Hill Village has generated attention for its successful attempt to help the elderly stay in their own homes. People like Miriam Huggard, a frail ninety-three-year-old who had lived in Boston for about fifty years, might have been forced into an ALF or a nursing home without it. She needed some help for some activities of daily living and looked into assisted living. It seemed to her "like a pretty good system." But she could not bear to leave the home in which she had lived so long.

The Beacon Hill Project, a nonprofit group, was responsive to her needs. The project now has 340 members aged fifty-two to ninety-eight. For $550 a year it provides weekly grocery deliveries, referral services, and volunteers who check regularly on her. In addition, it provides discounts on such services as housekeeping. And if a health care aide is needed, Beacon Hill Village can find one for eighteen dollars an hour.[4]

Susan McWhinney-Morse, seventy-two, president of Beacon Hill Village and a founder of the association, described its vision: "We wanted everything you'd find in a retirement community or assisted living—but we wanted these services in our own homes. We didn't want to leave the neighborhood we love." The association itself is run by Judy Willett, a social worker, who has two other employees. She said that they have never had a request they couldn't handle—including a resident's call from the hospital asking for a pickup of betting slips from the track.[5]

The reality is that most elderly persons do not live either in assisted living facilities, nursing homes, or other "institutions" specifically designed for them. Only 11 percent of the elderly live in such places. The rest live at home. By 2030 there will be about 63 million elderly living at home.[6]

OF NORCS AND SUPPORTIVE SERVICE PROGRAMS

The building in which I live is special to me. But as a naturally occurring retirement community, it is not unique in North America. Indeed, NORCs exist in some profusion. One estimate reported five thousand apartment houses identified as NORCs in the United States. In May 2002 the federal government began its National NORC Demonstration Project, a study of five cities—Baltimore, Cleveland, Pittsburgh, Philadelphia, and St. Louis—to determine how the elderly can be helped to remain in their own homes.[7]

The largest such community is Co-op City in the Bronx, New York—home to about 8,000 residents over sixty-five and 22,000 under that age. They reside in a number of buildings containing a total of 15,000 units. Co-op City was built in the 1960s as a model of "affordable housing at a price you can afford . . . for the family with children . . . covering 300 acres (200 city blocks)." The first of thirty-five buildings was opened in 1968, when a one-bedroom apartment sold for $1,350. In 2003 that apartment sold for under $6,000. But buyers could not have an income under $18,000 or over $100,000.[8]

Maintenance fees are also controlled. A resident who bought a seven-room apartment for $2,000 paid a monthly maintenance fee of $500 in 2002. Co-op City remains populated by middle-income residents, such as mail carriers and taxi drivers.

Many residents raised families in the large Co-op City complex. Children grew to adulthood and moved on. But many of their parents stayed. This was their home; they knew their neighbors, and this was affordable housing (in no small measure subsidized by the state and local governments). It was also housing in need of substantial repair, and money was in short supply.

Co-op City had become a naturally occurring retirement community. But it was one in need of special services if it was to survive. New York City's United Hospital Fund started the Aging in Place Initiative to meet the needs not only of Co-op City but other NORCs in the area. Fredda Vladeck, director of the program, said it was seen as a challenge and an opportunity. Funding for the program has come from local and state governments and also from foundation support and minimal charges to residents.

In 2002 Co-op City received a NORC budget of $1.2 million, which paid for forty personnel—including two nurses and four social workers—to provide support for elderly residents and allow Co-op City to function as an apartment complex. That support includes helping a husband whose wife suffers from Alzheimer's stay in their unit without recourse to a nursing home. It means, as well, preventive health courses in nutrition and medications. And it includes activities, both in and outside the complex. In fact, some residents who sold their units and moved into nursing homes later attempted to buy back into the complex, hoping to return to their life among friends.

Co-op City, like many large residential complexes, is run by a management company under contract with the resident owners' association. "We would be stranded without the NORC program," said one of the management officers. "We're not doctors. We're not social workers. We're real estate managers. We needed these programs to come in."[9]

According to Vladeck, the NORC program creates partnerships with social service and medical providers as well as real estate management organizations. She wrote:

> NORCs are housing developments or neighborhoods which were built for families but which, over time, have evolved into communities with a significant proportion of households headed by seniors. A number of NORCs have recognized that this intense aging in place of their residents both provides a challenge to the quality of life for individual seniors and their community and, because of population density, an opportunity to organize efficient and effective services to address their needs. A NORC supportive service program (SSP) is developed in response to this challenge and can help enable seniors to remain living in their own homes as they grow older and more frail.
>
> Programs are organized on site and include a full range of both preventive and supportive services which include: social and recreational programs; traditional social services; information and referral; case assistance and case management; health promotion; monitoring; chronic care management; and, increasingly, mental health services. Depending on the particular needs of a community, additional services may be organized such as transportation, laundry and shopping, etc.
>
> They serve the full range of seniors living in the community and, through their work, are often responsible for the reweaving of the social fabric of that community. Volunteers are critical to the program. Partnerships are central to the ethos of the SSP. Governance is shared by service providers, housing management, and community residents, while services are provided by a consortium of agencies, often drawing on each other's professional strengths. Funding is also through collaboration of public and private sources—local and, in some instances, state government support, philanthropic funds, and some user fees (usually modest contributions for the classes or activities programs).[10]

HOME CARE: A CAVEAT

Living in one's own home and neighborhood, receiving skilled care by people of one's choosing, and being helped by the government when needed: this mix seems to serve the best interests of individuals, their families, and government. Individuals then retain substantial control over their lives and keep their homes; their families have a certain measure of security in knowing that parents have access to skilled care when needed; and the government saves enormous sums.

Many of the people helped would otherwise be eligible for nursing homes at an annual cost to government of up to $65,000. From 1992 to 2002, the number of those covered by waiver programs has tripled to eight hundred thousand. More than half of these individuals are over sixty-five. The program cost during the same period went from $2 billion to $15 billion. (If her doctor had approved, my mother would have been covered by a waiver program, which would have permitted full-time help in her assisted living apartment at Glengrove.)

But there is a caveat to the remedy of home care, which often is funded largely by the federal government, as a waiver to Medicaid, and provided in defined programs by states: How is that care monitored to ensure that the services paid for are in fact delivered in a proper way?

Investigators from the U.S. General Accounting Office in 2003 examined fifteen of the largest waivers in fifteen states. A total of 266,700 elderly persons were to have received services under the waivers. The investigators found problems with the quality of care in eleven of the programs. In many cases, the services paid for simply had not been delivered. (In 2002, $258 billion was spent on Medicaid. The federal share was 57 percent.)

The federal administrator of the Centers for Medicare and Medicaid Services said he was not aware of the extent of the problem. He claimed that, in any event, it was the responsibility of the states to ensure "quality assurance." But he was not about to order federal investigators to enter people's homes as enforcers.[11]

Where does that leave individuals? It leaves them to their own devices to complain and delve into the bureaucracy to seek remedies—a not altogether pleasant prospect. An editorial in the *New York Times* warned that "the lack of oversight raises the frightening possibility that the nation could be headed into another social experiment that starts with great promise and ends with human disasters. . . . Congress will need to make sure that home care and independent living really work for the patients, not just for the budgeteers."[12]

A promising approach in eldercare programs is now becoming a part of some employee benefit packages. These programs allow for such help as a geriatric nurse's home safety assessment, which might otherwise cost an employee between $300 and $400. (Recall, this is the kind of help my mother refused. I hope to be more accepting.)

Interestingly, on the face of it, these programs, unlike other broad-ranged health plans, seem to offer business benefits that exceed costs. In the United States, business loses about $11 billion a year because of absenteeism, turnover, and lost productivity among full-time employees who care for elderly people, according to a 1997 study by the MetLife Mature Market Institute and the National Alliance for Caregiving. Adult children who live within an hour of their parents' homes are among the most affected. The National Council on Aging reported that about a quarter of such workers caring for their parents tend to miss work at least one day each month.

Under U.S. law, workers employed by companies of fifty or more employees may take up to twelve weeks of unpaid leave to care for immediate family members who have a serious health condition. The fact is, however, that very few workers seem to take advantage of such eldercare programs. The estimate is that no more than 5 percent of those covered by eldercare (about fifteen million) actually use the benefit package. At Ford, with a workforce of 165,000 protected by eldercare, during the first eighteen months of the program, only 147 made use of home safety assessments, although 1,600 employees had telephone consultations with geriatric specialists.

At times, the advice provided by such specialists can forestall an adult child's overreaction. Robert L'Hommedieu, eighty-one, suffered a serious fall on his snow-covered driveway in Pleasant

Valley, Missouri. His son, William, fifty-seven, thought that perhaps it was time to consider a nursing home. Instead, however, through his Ford eldercare benefit program, a geriatric nurse made a detailed home evaluation. The conclusion was that his father could safely continue in his home with a few modifications such as a shower—rather than a tub—and a med-alert button.

L'Hommedieu may not have been able to stay at home until his death, but with the help of a son who lived about five minutes from his father's home, he was able to stay there for several more years.[13]

SOME CLOSING THOUGHTS

I did not intend this narrative to be a memoir, although it has centered on the story of my mother's life at Glengrove. In a sense, it has been my story as well. My purpose has been to indicate choices we can make with our parents and for ourselves in planning and living in old age. It is also a story about the limits of choice, and the reality that no matter what option we choose, it cannot be perfect and cannot give us full control.

Often my mother accepted my help. Often she refused it. That refusal, and my own concerns and sense of duty as a son, led me to encourage her to move into an assisted living facility. In some ways I regret that decision. But I'm not sure that, even if I'd asked more questions and been more prepared, I would have urged her to make a different decision. At that time and in that place, assisted living seemed to be the best option for her.

Frailty, so the data indicate, does not necessarily come with old age, though the statistics relating to Alzheimer's disease certainly aren't encouraging. But I know that as I grow older, I might be in need of help with "activities for daily living."

If I need such help, I want to be the person making decisions. I want to choose the conditions for such help and the persons who will provide it. In effect, I want control over my life, and this includes control over my death. Control is a signal way to recognize the individual. I do not want—and I don't think most of us want—to be simply a body that health care givers, even with the best of intentions, treat as they think best.

Something else comes with control, something unique to the individual: *hope*. I am reminded again of Bertha, the quadriplegic chronic care hospital patient who had what seemed to be a permanent scowl. She had the use of only a single finger, but a recreation therapist showed her that she could use that finger to create mosaics—art of her own. And with the use of that finger came hope.

Marcie told the story of an elderly lady who brought her adult son to rent an apartment at my building. The son was suffering from AIDS. He had only a short time to live, but he wanted an apartment, a home of his own, one that he could plan. And plan he did. Shortly before he was to move into his new home, he died. His mother visited Marcie and told her how happy her son had been, planning his new home. He knew death was waiting, but even as it approached, he had hope.

I wish I had been able to give my mother that same hope. She deserved it. All of us deserve it.

Selecting an ALF: A Checklist

The following list summarizes key considerations that this book addresses relating to selecting an ALF. It assumes that an initial decision has been made for a parent to live his or her remaining days in an assisted living facility.

The list is addressed to you, an adult child. At this point, neither you nor your parent has given final approval to that decision. While your parent (usually your mother) will turn to you for advice—indeed, for the final decision—you should encourage her to give you as much input as she can. Choosing an ALF should be done thoughtfully and with patience, after thorough consideration of the issues in this list.

It's important to understand that, regardless of the smiles of the ALF's staff, the well-appointed decor, and even the welcome from residents your mother knows, this cannot be an impulse purchase (as I and so many other reasonably intelligent adults treated it). Once your mother becomes a resident, bonding with other residents, the staff, and the institution will occur within a short period. The decision to take up residence at the ALF will be difficult to change and is most likely a permanent one; it would be traumatic for your mother to leave her new home.

☐ Obtain the current tenancy contract and list of rules relating to residence. Read them carefully. Make an appointment (probably with the residence manager) to get your questions answered. *Never sign the contract after viewing the facility only once.*

☐ Ask if you and your mother might stay at the ALF for two days, one of which should be a Saturday or Sunday since this is a time when fewer staff are likely to be on duty. During your stay, take part in meals and activities. This will give you a sense of what life at the facility is like. And, of course, use the time to talk with staff members and other residents.

☐ Ask to visit the skilled health care unit. When first taking up residence in an ALF, the unit is not likely to evoke anxiety or fear. Later, following the first hospitalization (which almost always will occur), residents may be very fearful about admission to the unit. Now is a good time to have a tour, meet the staff, and ask the following questions:

- How many registered nurses are on duty at any particular time?
- Does the facility have a geriatric nurse practitioner on staff?
- Is there a training program for care aides?
- What is the staff turnover rate?
- Is there a physical therapist on staff? What is his or her role: Is it simply supervisory or will the physical therapist treat a resident who has returned from the hospital and lost strength and muscle mass?
- Is there a recreational therapist on staff?

Ask how decisions are made as to when a resident may return to her apartment following a stay in the unit.

☐ How are medical emergencies handled? Ask specific questions. How does the ALF deal with a fall, the most frequent kind of injury for residents? Under what circumstances is 911 called? What kind of continuing role, if any, will the ALF assume relating to monitoring and the care of the resident?

Does the ALF have a liaison with hospital staff to provide on-going communication with the resident's family?

☐ What is the ALF's policy as to a resident's end of life? If she is bedridden and given only limited time to live, will she be able to stay in her apartment? Will a properly recognized hospice be allowed to tend to her needs? First, discuss these matters with your mother, and be sure you fully understand her views. Then have a discussion with the manager of the ALF. Ask how the ALF reconciles its general rule requiring residents to live independently with its expressed promise of a resident's right to live (and die) in place. If the ALF's policy is that a resident has the right to die in place, have the manager show you where that is stated in the contract. If the answer is "Well, you have my word for it," respond with "That's fine, but I would like a brief, simple written statement to that effect, signed by the CEO and attached to the contract." If the statement is not provided, you may have difficulty later on. (Remember that the turnover rate, even among ALF management, is high. The person who made the verbal promise today may not be there tomorrow.)

☐ Find out if the state regulatory authority has investigated complaints and issued reports concerning the ALF. If so, ask to see copies of such reports. Where state law allows, such reports can be requested. (See resources below.)

☐ How do residents express their concerns about the ALF? Is there a residents' association? What are its functions? Ask for some examples of its activities.

☐ Does the ALF have a policy relating to theft from residents? Is this a problem for the ALF? (This question will test the ALF manager's credibility. Theft is endemic in nearly all ALFs; it is a problem not easily solved. A candid answer will acknowledge that there is a problem. A denial will suggest that the manager is not being forthcoming.)

☐ Is there a mechanism for the residents' guarantors to have their concerns heard by senior management?

☐ Ask to see the charges for rent and services during the past five years. You may get some idea of a pattern of cost increases.

☐ You will be asked to give a financial statement as guarantor for your mother. Be candid. Ask for an interview with the ALF's financial officer for his or her opinion as to how long you can safely carry the costs incident to your mother's stay. Bear in mind, however, that the financial officer, at best, can give only an estimate that will not be binding on the ALF.

☐ Ask yourself whether you will have the patience to keep listening and negotiating, not just with the ALF staff but with your mother as her life enters a new and changing phase. Understand that there may be times when your patience is exhausted. Be prepared to back away, recharge, and reengage. To keep your balance, it helps to have a support group of friends, family and, yes, professionals.

RESOURCES

• A state-by-state regulatory summary of assisted living is available through the website of the National Center for Assisted Living (www.ncal.org; click on 2006 Assisted Living State Regulatory Review). The summary is written in lay language. You can scroll to the state of interest. The headings are essentially the same for each state: state agency contact (including address and phone number); ALF move in/move out requirements; resident assessments; and staffing requirements.

• The National Center for Assisted Living also provides an in-depth checklist (www.ncal.org; click on Consumer Information, then on "A Consumer's Guide to Assisted Living Facilities"). See also chapter 7 of this book.

• There will be a continuing need for negotiation by the adult children, the resident, and ALF staff at all levels. The Harvard Negotiation Project helped to shape useful tools and programs in getting to yes. Two quite readable books are Roger Fisher and William Ury, *Getting to Yes: Negotiating Agreement Without Giving In* (New York: Penguin, 1981); and Roger Fisher and Scott Brown, *Getting Together: Building a Relationship That Gets to Yes* (Boston: Houghton Mifflin, 1988).

Notes

Introduction

1. See, for example, Robert L. Kane and Joan C. West, *It Shouldn't Be This Way: The Failure of Long-Term Care* (Nashville, TN: Vanderbilt University Press, 2005); David Barton Smith, *Reinventing Care: Assisted Living in New York City* (Nashville, TN: Vanderbilt University Press, 2003).

1. Choice

1. Susan B. Garland, "Faraway Relatives Turning to Geriatrics Experts," *New York Times*, January 19, 2003.
2. American Geriatrics Society et al., "Guideline for the Prevention of Falls in Older Persons," *Journal of the American Geriatrics Society* 49 (2001): 664–672; S. P. Baker et al., *The Injury Fact Book* (New York: Oxford University Press, 1992).
3. Bernadette Wright, "Assisted Living in the United States: Research Report," www.aarp.org/research/housing-mobility/assistedliving/assisted_living _in_the_united_states.html#philosophy (accessed January 31, 2006).
4. Ellyn Spragins, "Help for Elderly Parent Can Fray Family Ties," *New York Times*, November 3, 2002.
5. Catherine Hawes, Charles D. Phillips, and Miriam Rose, "High Service or High Privacy Assisted Living Facilities, Their Residents and Staff: Results from a National Survey," U.S. Dept. of Health and Human Services, 2000.
6. Ibid.
7. Kathleen Vickery, "Top 30 Assisted Living Chains," *Provider*, July 2000, p. 35.
8. Daniel Jay Baum, *Warehouses for Death: The Nursing Home Industry* (Don Mills, ON: Burns and MacEachern, 1977).
9. Georgina Gustin, "A Volatile Mix?" *New York Times*, March 16, 2003.
10. Amy Goldstein, "Assisted Living: Paying the Price," *Washington Post*, February 20, 2001.
11. Ibid.
12. *Assisted Living: Quality-of-Life and Consumer Protection Issues*, GAO/T-HEHS-99-111 (Washington, DC: General Accounting Office, 1999).

2. Moving Day

1. Quoted in Beth Witrogen McLeod, ed., *And Thou Shalt Honor: The Caregiver's Companion* (New York: Rodale Publishers, 2002), p. 14.

2. See also Ibid., pp. 14–15.

3. Paula Span, "Welcome to the Future," *Washington Post,* June 9, 2002.

4. Catherine Hawes, Charles D. Phillips, and Miriam Rose, "High Service or High Privacy Assisted Living Facilities, Their Residents and Staff: Results from a National Survey," U.S. Dept. of Health and Human Services, 2000, pt. 3, sec. C1, C2.

5. Linda Villarosa, "At Elders' Home, Each Day Is Valentine's Day," *New York Times,* June 4, 2002.

6. Jan Wong, "The Return of the Auschwitz Nightmare," *Globe and Mail* (Toronto), September 21, 2002.

7. "Seniors Sip," http://www.cbc.ca/insite/AS_IT_HAPPENS_TORONTO/2003/1/6.html.

8. Emily Yoffe, "A Visit to My Future," www.slate.com (accessed August 25, 2006).

9. Hawes, Phillips, and Rose, "High Service or High Privacy," pt. 7, sec. F.

10. Jessica McGurk, *Recruitment and Retention Strategies* (Fairfax, VA: Assisted Living Federation of America, 2000).

3. The Early Years at Glengrove

1. For how this is true of ALFs generally, see Catherine Hawes, Charles D. Phillips, and Miriam Rose, "High Service or High Privacy Assisted Living Facilities, Their Residents and Staff: Results from a National Survey," U.S. Dept. of Health and Human Services, 2000, pt. 3, sec. C; Andrew Goldstein/Eagan, "Better Than a Nursing Home?" *Time,* August 13, 2001, http://www.time.com/time/archive/preview/0,10987,1000517,00.html.

2. See also Linda Villarosa, "At Elders' Home, Each Day Is Valentine's Day," *New York Times,* June 4, 2002; Tina Adler, "Love Endures," *Washington Post,* January 28, 2003.

3. Edward Lewine, "Here, a Stud Is Someone with His Own Hair," *New York Times*, February 18, 2003.

4. Ibid.

5. See Assisted Living Project, "Assisted Living in New York State: A Summary of Findings," November 2001, pp. 13, 17, http://www.ltccc.org/papers/assisted_living_project.htm.

6. This is explored in Margaret Crowl, "Breaking in a New Boss: Have Your 'Spiel' Ready," *Plain Views, HealthCare Chaplains* 1, no. 23 (2005).

7. Ibid., pp. 459–467.

8. Jacquelyn Beth Frank, "How Long Can I Stay? Aging in Place in Assisted Living," *Journal of Housing for the Elderly* 15, no. 1/2 (2001).

4. The Staff and the Boss

1. Andrew Goldstein, "Better Than a Nursing Home?" *Time,* August 13, 2001, p. 44.
2. Catherine Hawes, Charles D. Phillips, and Miriam Rose, "High Service or High Privacy Assisted Living Facilities, Their Residents and Staff: Results from a National Survey," U.S. Dept. of Health and Human Services, 2000, pt. 7, sec. C.
3. Ibid.
4. Jessica McGurk, *Recruitment and Retention Strategies for Assisted Living Facilities* (Fairfax, VA: Assisted Living Federation of America Human Resources Executive Council, 2000).
5. Ibid.
6. Hawes, Phillips, and Rose, "High Service or High Privacy."
7. Ibid., sec. E(5).
8. Ibid., pt. 3, sec. C(1).
9. Ibid., sec. E(4).
10. Mr. Clegg to author, April 7, 2004; Graeme Smith, "Seniors Launch Rent Strike to Protest Loss of Alarms," *Globe and Mail,* March 2, 2004; Alison Mayes, "Angry Seniors Withhold Rent Cheques," March 2, 2004, www.fftimes.com.
11. "Woman, 86, on Hunger Strike over Care," April 27, 2005, www.cbc.ca.
12. Hawes, Phillips, and Rose, "High Service or High Privacy," pt. 3. sec. G.

5. Health

1. Ivan Illich, *Limits to Medicine—Medical Nemesis: The Expropriation of Health* (Toronto: McClelland and Stewart, 1976), pp. 273–275.
2. Catherine Hawes, Charles D. Phillips, and Miriam Rose, "High Service or High Privacy Assisted Living Facilities, Their Residents and Staff: Results from a National Survey," U.S. Dept. of Health and Human Services, 2000, pt. 3, sec. C(1).
3. Alzheimer's Association, "Glossary," www.alz.org/Resources/Glossary.asp.
4. Alzheimer's Disease Education and Referral Center, "Diagnosis: Alzheimer's Disease," www.alzheimers.org/diagnosis; N. R. Kleinfield, "More Than Death, Many Elderly Fear Dementia," *New York Times,* November 11, 2002; Gina Kolata, "Study Hints at Nongenetic Factors in Causing Alzheimer's," *New York Times,* February 14, 2001; Elaine Carey, "For Alzheimer's Day, Grim Stats, Fresh Hope," *Toronto Star,* September 21, 2004.
5. U.S. Center for Disease for Control, "Summary: Knowledge, Attitudes, and Practices of Physicians Regarding Urinary Incontinence in Persons Aged Greater Than or Equal to 65 Years—Massachusetts and Oklahoma, 1993," www.cdc.gov; see also L. S. Mitteness, "Knowledge and Beliefs about Urinary Incontinence in Adulthood and Old Age," *Journal of the American Geriatric Society* 38 (1990): 374–378.

6. Steve Lohr, "Bush's Next Target: Malpractice Lawyers," *New York Times*, February 27, 2005.

7. This is an unusually long time. See Peter Salgo, "The Doctor Will See You for Exactly Seven Minutes," *New York Times*, March 22, 2006.

8. For physician-patient communications see Gina Kolata, "When the Doctor Is In, but You Wish He Wasn't," *New York Times*, November 30, 2005.

9. Mary-Ellen Phelps-Deily, "For Seniors Balance Is Essential," *Washington Post*, October 16, 2001; N. R. Kleinfeld, "For Elderly, Fear of Falling Is a Risk in Itself," *New York Times*, March 5, 2003.

10. Hawes, Phillips, and Rose, "High Service or High Privacy," pt. 3, sec. E; "Elderly Stuck in Bed Limbo," *Toronto Star*, May 28, 2002.

11. "Errors That Kill Medical Patients," *New York Times*, December 18, 2002.

6. The End of My Mother's Life

1. The Nursing Home Reform Act is included in the Omnibus Reconciliation Act of 1987, *United States Code* 42, §§ 1395i-3 and 1936r et seq.; *Code of Federal Regulations* 42, pt. 483.

2. Lincoln Hospital, "Long Term Care," http://lincolnhospital.org/long_term_care.htm.

7. Assisted Living Can Succeed

1. Robert L. Kane and Joan West, *It Shouldn't Be This Way: The Failure of Long-Term Care* (Nashville, TN: Vanderbilt University Press, 2005); Trudy Lieberman, "Nursing Homes: When a Loved One Needs Care" (Yonkers, NY: Consumer Reports, 1996); Bruce C. Vladeck, *Unloving Care: The Nursing Home Tragedy* (New York: Basic Books, 1980), p. 263.

2. Motoko Rich, "Eviction Threat Can Loom for Independent Elderly," *New York Times*, February 15, 2004.

3. Amy Goldstein, "Assisted Living: Helping Hand May Not Be Enough," *Washington Post*, February 19, 2001.

4. This proposal was suggested by a prominent U.S. surgeon in a letter to the author.

5. See chap. 6, note 2.

6. U.S. Bureau of Labor Statistics, *2003 Wage Data* and *2002–2012 Employment Projections*.

7. Jan Thayer, "Statement on Behalf of the National Center for Assisted Living, Federal Trade Commission/Department of Justice, Hearing on Long Term Care/Assisted Living," June 11, 2003, pp. 6–7.

8. Kane and West, *It Shouldn't Be This Way*.

9. National Center for Assisted Living, "Planning Ahead: A Consumer's Guide to Assisted Living Facilities," http://www.longtermcareliving.com/planning_ahead/assisted/assisted1.htm.

10. Harvard School of Public Health, 2005; U.S. Department of Health and

Human Services, Centers for Disease Control and Prevention, "National Diabetes Fact Sheet," Atlanta, GA, September 29, 2004.

11. N. R. Kleinfeld, "Living at the Epicenter of Diabetes, Defiance and Despair," *New York Times*, January 10, 2006; Ian Urbina, "In the Treatment of Diabetes, Success Often Does Not Pay," *New York Times*, January 11, 2006.

12. Eric Carlson, "In the Sheep's Clothing of Resident Rights: Behind the Rhetoric of Negotiated Risk in Assisted Living," National Senior Citizens Law Center, 2003, available online at www.nsclc.org.

13. Thayer, "Statement," p. 8.

8. For Ourselves

1. Jane Gross, "The Middle Class Struggles in the Medicaid Maze," *New York Times*, July 9, 2005.

2. Elizabeth Harris, "For Boomers Near Retirement, Toolboxes Aplenty," *New York Times*, January 4, 2004.

3. Barbara Basler, "Declaration of Independents: Home Is Where You Want to Live Forever," *AARP Bulletin*, December 2005, p. 14.

4. Barbara Whitaker, "These Days, 'Retirement Living' Can Mean Many Things," *New York Times*, February 6, 2006; Jane Gross, "Aging at Home: For a Lucky Few, a Wish Come True," *New York Times*, February 9, 2006.

5. Gross, "Aging at Home."

6. Alan Feuer, "Haven for Workers in Bronx Evolves for Their Retirement," *New York Times*, August 5, 2002.

7. Ibid.

8. Erica Pearson, "Troubles for Co-op City and Middle Class Housing in NYC," *Gotham Gazette*, October 13, 2003, http://www.gothamgazette.com/article//20031013/200/555.

9. Feuer, "Haven for Workers."

10. Fredda Vladeck, personal communication, 2003.

11. Robert Pear, "Report Criticizes Federal Oversight of State Medicaid," *New York Times*, July 7, 2003.

12. "Is Home Care Really Working?" editorial, *New York Times*, July 8, 2003.

13. Maggie Jackson, "Companies Adding Benefits for Care of the Elderly," *New York Times*, July 7, 2002.

Index

nursing homes
    interface with ALFs, 151–52
    regulations covering, 151

orientation, in ALFs, 43–45, 161
ownership, of ALFs, 19–20

para-chaplaincy. *See* chaplaincy
physical therapists, role of, 128–30,
    132, 137
physicians
    malpractice liability, 106, 120
    power over ALF residents, 106
profile, of Americans entering ALFs, 3,
    17–18, 47

recreation therapists, role of, 137–38,
    163–64
regulation, government, of ALFs, 159
rent subsidy programs, 94–95
rents, 3, 18, 21–23
    discretion of ALF management to de-
        termine, 159
    increases, 89–90
    resisting increases, 90–92, 95

residents' associations, role of, 61–64,
    159

safety, in the home, 13–15
satisfaction scores, ALF residents, 70
security, 71–73
services
    discretion of ALF management to de-
        termine fees, 159
    examples of, 35–36
    fee increases, 89–90
    resisting fee increases, 90–92, 95
sexual intimacy, in ALFs, 56–58
social workers, in ALFs, role of, 161–
    62

theft, in ALFs, 80–83
turnover, of ALF CEOs, 87
turnover, of ALF staff
    effect on residents, 46, 75, 77
    national rates of, 45

unions, in ALFs, role of, 82–84

volunteers, role of, 64–66, 125–26